FLOATING

IN THE

DEEP END

ALSO BY PATTI DAVIS

Homefront, 1986

Deadfall, 1988

The Way I See It, 1992

Bondage, 1994

Angels Don't Die, 1995

Two Cats and the Woman They Own, 1996

The Long Goodbye, 2004

The Lives Our Mothers Leave Us, 2009

Till Human Voices Wake Us, 2013

The Wit and Wisdom of Gracie (A Pug's Guide to Life), 2014

The Earth Breaks in Colors, 2014

The Wrong Side of Night, 2019

FLOATING
IN THE
DEEP END

How Caregivers Can See
Beyond Alzheimer's

WITHDRAWN

Patti Davis

LIVERIGHT PUBLISHING CORPORATION

A Division of W. W. Norton & Company

Independent Publishers Since 1923

Copyright © 2021 by Patti Davis
Foreword copyright © 2021 by Mary Catherine Mayo

All rights reserved
Printed in the United States of America
First Edition

For information about permission to reproduce selections from this book, write to Permissions, Liveright Publishing Corporation, a division of W. W. Norton & Company, Inc., 500 Fifth Avenue, New York, NY 10110

For information about special discounts for bulk purchases, please contact W. W. Norton Special Sales at specialsales@wwnorton.com or 800-233-4830

Manufacturing by LSC Communications
Production manager: Julia Druskin

Library of Congress Cataloging-in-Publication Data

Names: Davis, Patti, author.
Title: Floating in the deep end : how caregivers can see beyond Alzheimer's / Patti Davis.
Description: First edition. | New York, NY : Liveright Publishing Corporation, [2021]
Identifiers: LCCN 2021025725 | ISBN 9781631497988 (hardcover) | ISBN 9781631497995 (epub)
Subjects: LCSH: Alzheimer's disease. | Alzheimer's disease—Patients—Care. | Caregivers. | Fathers and daughters.
Classification: LCC RC523 .D376 2021 | DDC 616.8/311—dc23
LC record available at https://lccn.loc.gov/2021025725

Liveright Publishing Corporation, 500 Fifth Avenue, New York, N.Y. 10110
www.wwnorton.com

W. W. Norton & Company Ltd., 15 Carlisle Street, London W1D 3BS

1 2 3 4 5 6 7 8 9 0

*This book is dedicated to Dr. David Feinberg,
in appreciation for his support and confidence in
Beyond Alzheimer's. I am eternally grateful.*

Contents

Foreword

By Mary Catherine Mayo, MD

In writing *Floating in the Deep End*, and before that in bringing into being Beyond Alzheimer's, a support group for caregivers, Patti Davis has taken an incredibly difficult personal experience and galvanized it into a years-long mission to provide knowledge, support, guidance, and reassurance to Alzheimer's caregivers. As a caregiver for her father, she did extensive work and research in the care of Alzheimer's patients and learned a great deal of practical knowledge. She also tapped into the specific needs and challenges faced by those *providing care* to Alzheimer's patients, including their important spiritual journey. I had the privilege of being a part of Beyond Alzheimer's as a cofacilitator with Patti and was frequently awed by her kindness, humor, and compassion.

There is a saying in medicine, "See one, do one, teach one." The phrase typically refers to learning a procedure and then passing along this knowledge, but it comes to mind here as well. Through her

insight and perspective, Patti, in the pages that follow, provides guidance, reassurance, and a sense of connection to others experiencing
various stages of caring for loved ones with dementia and the unique
feelings that come with being overwhelmed and alone. Patti, through
this book as well as by establishing the support group, has not only
provided much-needed advice for various specific challenges during
this time but also has enabled caregivers to forge connections and
obtain much-needed support.

Upon meeting a new patient with memory concerns, a physician's initial role is to diagnose and treat. While there are some
treatments for symptoms of such patients, there is a lack of disease-
altering medications for dementia. Exercise, good nutrition and
sleep habits, among other lifestyle adjustments, are encouraged, but
above all the goal is to ensure the safety and happiness of the patient.
Together with the family, medical professionals aim to identify and
address potential risks for a patient, and to ensure safety at each
stage of disease progression. It is, most of the time, an incredible
burden for a family member to approach, and the specific challenges
continue to evolve over time. And while no two patients are alike,
there are similarities and common experiences among patients with
dementia and their caregivers. As patients lose cognitive abilities,
they often begin to feel more and more untethered to the buoy that
once was their identity. And overworked caregivers, who assume the
role of the life raft, can feel as if they are sinking altogether.

Caregiver burnout is nearly unavoidable in supporting a patient
with dementia, at least at some point during the course of a loved
one's disease. Beyond Alzheimer's helps so many to not feel quite
so alone. Providing this support is an invaluable resource not only
for caregivers but the patients themselves, as they directly benefit

as well. Patti has a particular ability to find the blessings and teachings in the smallest of moments, and it was both an honor as well as wonderfully touching to witness her inherent intuition and empathy. This book is a rare and special gift Patti has provided for us all by opening up about her experiences and by sharing her knowledge, so that even more families struggling with this difficult journey may find some solace.

Introduction

In the end, we remember people in pieces—slivers of memory, images, bursts of sound, and trails of whispers. When I remember my father, I think of his eyes. As a child, I searched for them, wanting feverishly for them to focus on me, twinkle as they always did when he was about to say something funny or indulge one of my childish fantasies, like searching for leprechauns when the moon was full. On bright California days his eyes seemed to match the sky. But I remember also how they could take on a mineral stillness when he was determined to teach me something important, like getting back on my horse after I fell off.

I remember his shoulders, broad enough for me to sit on when I was small, strong enough to hoist me up onto a horse, build fences at our ranch. His legs were a swimmer's legs, lean and sinewy. He had perfect form when executing a dive into the pool, and his kicks when he swam were hard and athletic. When I was a child, I used to say that my father could do anything. My parents found it cute, so I said it often. But I meant it; I thought nothing could get the best of him. A lifetime later, I would watch him stand helplessly in front of a beast he could not slay.

When Alzheimer's began stealing him away, his eyes were my barometer for how quickly, how relentlessly, the disease was progressing. In the early stages they reached for what was still recognizable, sinking back into fear if what had once been familiar suddenly was not. At some point during the ten years of his illness, he was pirated to a place far away, and the only comfort was that his eyes looked relaxed, as if it was okay to be there. Over time, they changed color, fading from blue to an uncertain shade of gray, like the sky when fog drifts across it. A week or so before he died, he closed his eyes and I thought they would probably never open again. But they did.

The night before he died, the nurse unbuttoned his pajama top to listen to his heart through the stethoscope. His shoulders were so thin, just edges of bone and pale skin. I rested my hand around his left shoulder; it fit into the curve of my palm. Then I asked the nurse if I could listen to his heartbeat. She handed me the stethoscope.

"It's weak," she said. "Thready."

I heard it like an echo. A heart that was leaving this world. A heart I had always wanted to know better, to feel closer to. I knew I'd remember the sound for the rest of my days.

Seconds before my father died, his eyes opened. They were bright blue and focused, twinkling like they once did so long ago, in a time that seemed like ancient history. He focused on my mother, let his eyelids fall again, and in an instant he was gone.

≈

IN 1994, THE YEAR my family's life changed forever, people were not talking about Alzheimer's. When my father released his letter to the country and the world revealing he had been diagnosed with the disease, the Reagans suddenly became the poster family for an illness no one wanted to discuss. I was living in Manhattan at the time, and if ever I was recognized on the street strangers would often stop me and mention his Alzheimer's. Usually they would say that they were praying for him, or that they were so sorry this had happened. But occasionally someone would share a snippet of personal experience with a loved one who had been given the same diagnosis. It would always be brief, almost cryptic—an image through a half-open window. And then they'd be gone. I was left with glimpses into their experience, never the full story.

I remember walking along Columbus Avenue one drizzly afternoon after such an encounter and realizing that I needed to accept the fact that I was alone on a journey I knew nothing about. I felt as though I was embarking on a trek through the Himalayas without a Sherpa. I knew there would be stumbles and times I would feel lost, but I committed myself to embracing the passage of my father's exit from this world, whatever that would mean.

Obviously, my siblings and my mother were on this journey as well. But the stark truth about Alzheimer's is that everyone loses the person who is ill in their own way, according to the architecture of their relationship with that individual. My brothers, my sister, and certainly my mother were going to lose my father in ways that were different from my loss. Even in a family that's close and communicative it's still a pilgrim's path, and the loneliness settles deep in your bones.

ALMOST FROM THE START, I thought about the mysteries of memory, and how we are shaped and guided by what we remember of our experiences, our history, our life lessons. All these things imprint us, mold us into the person we eventually become. So what is left if our memory is whittled away? Are we just empty vessels, a collection of cells with no identity? Some deep part of me couldn't accept that, and what came to me was the belief that would ground me during the years ahead: I didn't believe a person's soul could have Alzheimer's. I made the decision that if I kept reaching beyond the disease, if I kept aiming for my father's soul, I would somehow be able to connect with him. Or I'd at least have a chance at connecting. It would, without question, be an exercise in faith.

I realize some might read this and think that this isn't for them, that as an atheist or agnostic they don't believe in the soul being a separate entity. I am not here to proselytize; other people's belief systems are none of my business. I would simply ask you to consider the possibility. You don't know that it's not true, and if you are facing the challenge of a loved one with any form of dementia, you're going to need all the tools you can get.

Antoine de St. Exupéry said, "It is only with the heart that one can see rightly. What is essential is invisible to the eye." I came upon that quote shortly after my father's diagnosis, and for the many years that he spent leaving this world in stages, I held onto it like a mantra, determined to see with my heart what was invisible to my eyes.

I didn't know what to expect from Alzheimer's—no one does, because every individual is different—but I knew that language would fail, that memories would turn to ash, and that no new memories would be formed. Still I kept believing that a perfectly intact soul rested in the mysterious realm beyond cognitive thought.

My father had always seemed larger than life to me, yet he carried distance with him, as if it had been encoded in his DNA. As far back as childhood, long before the glare of the world's spotlight, I sensed a mystery about him, something out of reach that made it seem as if his path on this earth was wide and important, as though he were here for far weightier tasks than parenting me.

When I was in the sixth grade he helped me build a science project on the human heart. I remember sitting beside him in the yard, the fall air sharp and cool around us, as he patiently assembled a plastic replica, complete with clear tubes for the arteries and red-dyed water for blood. As the heart came together, I wondered about his and why I couldn't get closer to it. Looking back now, I think all of us had a sense that the world was beckoning him, and he was eager to answer the call. This was one thing I had in common with my siblings—we all longed to know him better, despite the sad resignation of instinct that we never would.

With Alzheimer's, he seemed to grow smaller. Everyone with the disease does; it's one of the few constants in an otherwise unpredictable illness. Holding on to the belief that his soul was unaffected allowed me to not get lost in the diminishment of his physical being. I saw it, mourned what was being stolen, but I clung to the confidence that his soul was deep, fathomless, and no illness could intrude upon it.

I didn't know it then, but the seeds were being planted for the support group program I would start many years later, a group for caregivers and family members of people with dementia. The program I would call Beyond Alzheimer's.

After my father died, I thought for a while that my time with Alzheimer's was over, that its hold on me had been broken and I would look back on it as a chapter of my life—one in which I had changed and grown. I didn't see it as an experience that would chart the course of my life going forward in many ways.

How naïve of me, I think now.

WHAT HAPPENED WAS, other eyes started to tug at me. They were the eyes of strangers who would occasionally stop me in grocery stores or on the sidewalk. They would share with me personal details of what they were going through with Alzheimer's (or one of the other versions of dementia). They would tell me about a father or a mother, sometimes a spouse, who they could no longer reach, who no longer knew them, who had either gradually or suddenly stopped recognizing them. Sometimes their eyes brimmed with tears, other times their eyes were wide and unblinking, as if they were too exhausted to cry. Always, they seemed haunted. Alzheimer's drifts in through an unlocked door and proceeds to steal what is most valuable—a human being. You're helpless against it. You have no choice but to accept that you're its prisoner too.

I started to notice that when I listened to people who I didn't know and might never see again, when I offered some insights or realizations from my years with Alzheimer's, their eyes changed. Often it was just a slight shift, a leaning away from despair toward something that felt like hope. Hope that the prison walls weren't as solid as they seemed, hope that dementia wasn't the whole story—that there were hidden chambers past their loved one's ruined memory and broken language where the person they once knew could still be glimpsed. One woman, in the cereal aisle at Whole Foods, started crying and said, "Thank you. I haven't let myself cry enough. It's all bottled up in me." I had told her to not listen to the unlinked words her mother was uttering ("word salad," it's come to be called) but listen instead to the rise and fall of her voice, the tone, the emotional waves beneath the words. She probably still wouldn't know exactly what her mother was trying to communicate, but she'd get the emotional underpinnings and from those she could fashion a response.

"Sometimes it helps if you don't look at her," I told the woman. "Look away and just absorb her voice."

The way I came to that discovery is quirky and a bit unusual. One day, when I was intensely focused on my father, trying and failing to understand what he was saying, a memory popped into my mind. Many years earlier, in the eighties, I had spent an evening with John Belushi and Dan Ackroyd in New York. John abandoned us early, and Dan and his girlfriend drove me back to their apartment. At one moment in their living room he was talking about something (I don't remember what now) but I couldn't figure out if he was joking or serious.

I said to his girlfriend, "How do you know when he's joking?"

"Oh, it's easy," she told me. "Just don't look at him."

That memory stayed with me and it surfaced right when I needed it. It was how I figured out that if I didn't look at my father, the clues to what he was trying to say would be there in the cadence of his voice.

As lonely as my odyssey with Alzheimer's was, I'm actually grateful for the solitariness of the journey. I got to map things out for myself with no one telling me I was wrong, or crazy, or off base. Since people weren't talking about the disease, there was no temptation to call someone and say, for example, "I made this great discovery based on an evening I spent with Dan Ackroyd a long time ago. What do you think?" I can only imagine what the reaction would have been. But the truth was, when I trusted my instinct, when I relied on that particular memory and put it into practice, it worked.

Occasionally a stranger would slip in something about a parent who didn't have Alzheimer's but was the caregiver and mentioned how difficult that was. The comments were usually punctuated by long sighs, telegraphing exhaustion and exasperation. I would think afterward about how complicated it could sometimes be with my mother during the decade of my father's illness. I wanted to be a daughter who knew how to comfort, offer solace—my mother was, after all, losing the love of her life. But the language of my family was one of distance and fractures and trepidation. I had to learn a new language and try it out in an environment where it might not be accepted. My mother had frightened me for my entire life; I would have to reach past that fear in order to offer comfort. There were moments when I think I got it right, but there were many other times when fear stopped me.

Ultimately, I learned another important lesson: as much as Alzheimer's, and the person who has it, comes to dominate your life, it also presents you with an opportunity to free yourself from the domination of the past. The dynamics that were once in place don't need to define the future. I'd spent so many decades longing for what I was never going to get from my parents. Alzheimer's made me realize that I had to be the one to change. A friend of mine told me how she had been regaling her therapist with all the ways she had tried and was still trying to elicit tenderness from her mother—a woman who had never shown any. The therapist finally said to her. "Why do you keep going to the hardware store for bread?" It was a brilliant description of what many of us do. I resolved to stop looking for what I wasn't going to find and pay close attention to what was there.

By 2001 I had been doing lectures for several years. At events and various gatherings I spoke about being the daughter of someone with Alzheimer's and what I was learning from the experience. I had a lecture date in Michigan booked for mid-September, which had been set many months earlier. Then 9/11 happened. As a nation we were driven to our knees, numb with shock and ragged with grief. I remember, as we all do, the silent skies and the pall of sadness everywhere. I had no idea if planes would start flying again in time for my lecture, and frankly I was kind of hoping they wouldn't. Not only did I not want to get on a plane, I didn't know how to fit in the devastation we were all going through with the subject matter I was expected to talk about. And I felt I had to include it. I couldn't ignore what was uppermost in everyone's thoughts. As it turned out, planes did resume flying a couple of days before my lecture date.

The talk I gave, so soon after the towers fell, focused more on grief than I had in other lectures. And then I brought up the question that was gripping all of us: Why? Why was such unimaginable evil sent our way? Why were those who died in the towers, or in the planes, present at that time when there were other people who, at the last minute, stopped for coffee, or took a day off, or changed flights, and lived because of that one small choice? Why does a good, kind person get Alzheimer's when someone down the road who is mean and dishonest and yells at the neighborhood kids is enjoying perfect health? Where is the sense in all this, or is it all just random? I told those who had come to listen to me that I had no answer for any of those questions, and people much wiser than I don't have answers either. It's a question that can never be answered, not on this side of life anyway. A far better question is: What can I learn from this? If you say to yourself, I don't understand this, I can't make sense out of it, but I'm willing to be open to whatever lessons are folded into this situation, then you change your experience of the experience, at least in small ways.

It seemed to register with the people I was speaking to, and I realized I was also saying it to try to keep myself on a path of learning and staying open. I needed to reinforce it in myself. It's not easy when life slams into you and you find yourself struggling through grief. It's hard to let go of asking why, of trying to make sense out of what makes no sense. With Alzheimer's, with a devastating experience like 9/11, with any overwhelming tragedy, there are no visible markers to guide us through the fog. When pilots can't see where they're going because of clouds or fog, they rely on instruments. We have internal instruments—strengths we didn't realize we had, insights, faith, all of which can help pull us through. That lecture date has stayed with me not only because of when it was but because I looked out at people with their arms around a companion, or maybe a stranger—I couldn't be sure—and I thought about the sweetness of grief and how it can heal us in times of great wound and stunning loss. I looked out at faces that were streaked with tears but that had a resolve, a determination to go on despite the pain.

It was a lesson in the power and beauty of shared sorrow. A group of people came out to listen to someone else's experience with a disease that had upended their lives. I learned from the question-and-answer portion about the young mother whose father couldn't remember from one visit to the next who the little baby was that his daughter was holding. She wanted her father to be able to hold his grandson, but she was too afraid he would drop the baby. I learned about the wife whose husband no longer recognized her, and the man who now bathed his father in the tub, talking to him as if he were a child. Everyone there had a story that they carried with them, woke up to each morning, and wept over most nights. And then there was the bigger story linking us all. Planes into the towers, thousands of people dead on a bright blue morning, a day that made us wonder if hate was winning and if we would ever heal.

What I saw in that crowd, on that day, was that the gentleness of grief was winning. I saw that while the details of everyone's story differed, their pain flowed from love.

IN THE TIME FOLLOWING my father's death, pulled by the words of strangers, I couldn't shake the feeling that my story wasn't unique. The wounds and scars in families can feel isolating until you realize you are part of a very large club—our stories are usually more alike than different. I knew there were countless caregivers wrestling with the same things I'd wrestled with. And while I learned a lot from the solitariness of my experience, I wanted to try to lessen the loneliness of others who were going through the same thing.

Someone once told me that there are two types of people in the world—those who go through a door and never turn around to see if someone's behind them, and those who hold the door open in case there is. I wanted to be in the latter category.

I'm not sure why it took me eight years after my father's death to start my support group, Beyond Alzheimer's. Maybe it simply took that long for me to organize within myself all that I had learned. Or it could be that I needed those years to recognize that once Alzheimer's enters your life, it never really leaves. For the decade of my father's illness, I felt as if I were floating in the deep end, tossed by waves, carried by currents, but not drowning. My lifelines were my faith and a stubborn resolve to look past the cruelty of the disease in order to learn from it.

At some point, I saw how Alzheimer's was actually enabling me to know my father a bit better. Apertures opened up. I got to see glimpses of the boy who raced into his house after school, pulled his ice skates out from under the bed, and skated on the river until the light started fading and his mother called to him from the back door. I got to see the athletic teenager who refused to let his acute near-sightedness hamper him. He was a lifeguard in the summers and rescued seventy-seven people (a fact that not even Alzheimer's could remove from his memory). I got to see the young man who dreamed of a bigger life than the one his parents had, who loved his father and learned tolerance and fairness from him, but who pledged to be nothing like him in other ways. Jack Reagan had long been a hostage to alcohol; success for him was always an out-of-reach dream sitting at the bottom of a whiskey glass. Alzheimer's moves a person back through time. If you're willing to follow them down that road, you learn things you might never have learned otherwise.

In 2011 I started the support group Beyond Alzheimer's at UCLA. I partnered with a cofacilitator from the medical field and ran it for five years there, then moved it to Saint John's Hospital in Santa Monica after there was an administrative change at UCLA. The group is now licensed at Geisinger Medical Center in Scranton, Pennsylvania, and Cleveland Clinic in Las Vegas, Nevada. My hope is that more hospitals will embrace the idea and offer the program to caregivers who need a safe place where they can talk freely and openly. Sadly, in the medical community there is still not enough of an investment in caring for the caregivers.

When I began the group I wasn't completely sure if the principles I'd come up with for myself would translate. During much of my father's illness when I lectured on the subject, audiences related to what I was saying, but I had learned more in the years since. I couldn't be certain that people coming to a support group would be on board with my approach. So, it was another leap of faith. But as the group continued, I started to see people find their footing in a landscape that was changing around them every day. My hope is that this book will do the same. It can't minimize or take away anyone's grief, but I hope it can light lamps on what is too often a very dark path.

This isn't a how-to book, although there certainly are suggestions along the way. Rather, it's an exploration of all the things that come up and sideline you as you live alongside this mysterious and relentless disease. Something that is not often made clear is that dementia is the category of disease for Alzheimer's and other variants. Each type of dementia has its own characteristics, which I will discuss, but the mystery and the pain of losing a loved one in this manner are the constants that unite everyone's experience. In this book, I use Alzheimer's and dementia interchangeably, and include all forms of the disease in what I'm describing unless I specify otherwise.

Often, in my support group I would suggest that instead of asking, "What should I do?" in a given situation, a better question is, "How should I be?" because that will ultimately determine what actions you take. Form always follows content. That doesn't mean that specific suggestions and methods aren't important—they are—and I will deal with many of them here. But as a caregiver your own emotional state is what influences the outcome.

When I started Beyond Alzheimer's I wanted it to be a support group that went deep, that delved into what was going on under the surface—the emotions that people hold tightly to and are reluctant to disclose. I don't know how you can possibly figure out how to handle the complex situations that Alzheimer's presents you with if you haven't taken a clear-eyed look at your family and what the dynamics are there, what the foundational history is. All of that is going to be magnified when Alzheimer's enters the picture.

Sometime after my father publicly announced that he had Alzheimer's there was a moment in which I thought maybe this might bring my family together. I know I'm not alone in having that hope. It's something that many people have expressed to me after such a serious diagnosis is made. I'm sorry to say this, but that tends to only work in movies and cheerful fairy tales where everyone lives happily ever after in the end. In real life, old wounds get exposed and stare you in the face. It's of course possible that dealing with those wounds might ultimately lead to newfound bonds within a family, but it doesn't happen the minute a terminal diagnosis is made.

It's interesting that just as there is a peeling away of layers in the person who has Alzheimer's, there is also a peeling away of layers in family members and loved ones. All of us develop protective layers to cover unresolved issues or old resentments; we do it to smooth things over in life, but we also do it to try to convince ourselves that we no longer have those issues or resentments. Enter Alzheimer's, and suddenly everything starts being exposed. It's both scary and illuminating to be confronted with things you either thought you'd dealt with or hoped you'd gotten rid of—how your mother or father treated you in the past, conflicts with siblings, dramas that weren't spoken about, divorces or addictions. Alzheimer's brings up everything. It's simply an aspect of the disease. But as with any experience, we always have a choice about how to respond.

In six years of running my support group, I can think of only three families who were strongly bonded to begin with and remained so once they learned that a family member had dementia. Siblings and the parent who was the primary caregiver would come to the group together and, even though there might be disagreements between them occasionally on what to do in certain circumstances, their bond of love and mutual respect was unbreakable. It was remarkable to see, and unfortunately rare. In most cases, families are like overly tilled ground—it's difficult to grow anything new there.

I don't think I ever stopped wishing that my family might figure out how to be a family. But it wasn't to be. Distance and dissonance had been our reality for too long; we didn't know any other way. There were efforts made in individual relationships. My sister Maureen and I started to speak often by phone when I was still living in New York, and whenever I flew back to see our father, we would get together. During that time, she was diagnosed with the melanoma that ultimately took her life, but even that couldn't change what was all too clear—we didn't have a strong foundation in my family. We were trying to build a house on sand. My brother Ron had built his own life in Seattle; he would visit sometimes but his life remained separate, unknown to the rest of us. My brother Michael kept running up against my mother's dislike of him, which was never going to lessen. And my mother and I were locked in the same complicated dance of coming together and then breaking apart. It was such an old pattern, it felt ancient and sadly predictable. It took me many years and a lot of work to unearth from my memory moments with my mother that were loving, even tender, and hold onto them as a vital part of our story.

I HAVE WATCHED PEOPLE who once felt shackled by the intrusion of dementia into their lives take a step back and change their focus. They learned to look at the disease differently and understand that it didn't have to steal their lives too. That meant reevaluating who they were choosing to be. What were they leading with, what were they holding onto? I have witnessed people accept their tears and their pain as tools, not punishment, and find strength in themselves that they didn't believe they had before.

I knew from my own experience where they were starting from, and where they could get to if they were determined enough. It's not an easy transition; it takes work, but it's possible. Several years before my father revealed his diagnosis, I had left California and moved to the East Coast. My marriage had failed, I had subsequently gotten into an abusive relationship, and I felt broken and useless. I did what I am prone to do. I ran away: I sold my house at the bottom of the market, I lost almost everything, and the spiral downward continued, seemingly without end. I could find no way out of the darkness. I was very seriously thinking about ending my life—the thought came to me every day, curling around me, whispering me awake at night. It was the second time in my life I had come to that edge, the first being when I was nineteen and threadbare from drugs. But this was different. This was the weight of a lifetime that I saw as a failure. I didn't know how to turn things around, and my soul felt exposed and exhausted.

Then I got the phone call saying my father was going to announce that he had Alzheimer's. I had been told by my brother Ron about the diagnosis some time before this, but I wasn't supposed to know. Neither was my father. I think the secrecy of it kept the whole thing feeling somewhat abstract. Suddenly, the disease and all it implied towered over my own pain. I remember the moment when something opened up in me and I decided to live. I had just hung up the phone, my mother's voice still echoing in my head, telling me that within the hour the world would know that my father had Alzheimer's. A shaft of sunlight was resting on my shoulder and Manhattan's street noise was coming in through the open window. I knew I needed to be there for my father's last passage. When the news hit that afternoon and I, along with America and the rest of the world, read his letter for the first time, I saw how he was going to embrace every moment that was left to him. If he could face the uncertainty of his remaining days with that kind of courage, I could look ahead with courage as well.

So, when people came into my support group with their broken places on full display, I knew what that pain felt like. And I knew if they kept coming into that room every week, where it was safe and supportive, where the group members listened to them and didn't judge, they could mend and transform and carve out a new way of living their lives. In a bizarre way, my father's Alzheimer's saved my life. It set me on a path to figuring out how I could be there for him through the blind curves of the disease. Ultimately, it inspired me to figure out how I could be there for others.

I never shared that dark chapter of my story with people in the support group. I have always believed that we intuitively know when another person can relate to what we are going through, and I trusted that they would know that about me. I decided to share it now because someone reading this might be on that same edge. Maybe they came to it by an accumulation of life's sorrows and fate's cruelties, maybe by a loved one's diagnosis of dementia. I want them to know that there is a way off that precipice, that even if Alzheimer's brought them there, it can also pull them back.

❧

THE UNDENIABLE TRUTH ABOUT losing a loved one to Alzheimer's is that you will not be the same person at the end of the journey as you were at the beginning. How you will be different, however, is a matter of choice. You will either be softer, more pliable, more open, or you will be harder, more brittle, more judgmental. It gets down to the choices you make every day. My goal in the work I have done, and with this book, is to encourage people to choose door #1. It's not only an easier way to go through life, but you will come to realize that, as counterintuitive as it seems, there are actually gifts folded into this disease. Grief is a powerful teacher if you allow it to be. It is both shadow and light, enemy and friend. It can pull you down to the murky river bottom, lift you above ancient battlefields, and often leave you hovering on air currents.

Alzheimer's, like any version of dementia, will undoubtedly bring chaos into your life. But in the midst of chaos, there are quiet spaces, moments of stillness, that wait for you to find them. Those spaces are where you are able to see beyond the wreckage of the disease, beyond all that you've lost, all that you miss, to an unfolding of new parts of yourself that were waiting for you to unearth them.

"In a dark time, the eye begins to see."

—THEODORE ROETHKE, "In a Dark Time"

THE WORLD JUST CHANGED

CHAPTER 1

The Diagnosis You Feared

It's almost never a surprise. By the time you take your loved one to the doctor to be evaluated and tested, there have usually been signs for a while. Interludes of confusion that are more pronounced than just temporary distraction or frayed strands of language. You may have noticed your loved one doesn't seem to recognize familiar people at first, or they're baffled when dealing with ordinary items around the house. Geography gets confusing; they tend to get lost, even in their own neighborhoods. One early warning sign can be that they've lost their sense of smell. Obviously, that can be caused by a cold or allergies, but if it persists for a long time, it should set off a few alarm bells. The sense of smell is intricately connected to brain function, and studies have shown that people who lose their sense of smell have an increased risk of getting dementia.[1]

Sometimes there are very few symptoms until the person either falls and suffers a head injury[2] or has to go under general anesthesia for a surgical procedure. Either of these two events can unleash dementia that has been lingering deep inside the brain. A head injury doesn't always result in dementia, although severe injuries can either cause or accelerate the disease. Anesthesia can reveal what has been lingering in the brain; suddenly there were symptoms where before there were none.[3]

The symptoms and the timing of dementia may vary, but the fear that arises in family members does not. The two most common responses from loved ones to seeking out a diagnosis are guilt and denial. Those who have gone ahead, made the necessary appointment, and received the diagnosis they feared often end up feeling guilty because they think they might have waited too long. If they had gone in sooner, they reason, their parent or relative or spouse wouldn't have wandered off that afternoon and ended up blocks away, not knowing where they were. Or that embarrassing episode at a restaurant might have been avoided. There is no upside to thinking like this, nor is there any logic. You did the best you could given the information you had. And the incidents you think would have been avoided might still have happened.

Dementia is a mysterious disease. It isn't like a melanoma, where you can physically see something on the skin that looks bad, something you can google and find pictures of, images that usually make it obvious you should get to a doctor. Symptoms of dementia show up but then seem to abate, and we all have a tendency to procrastinate when something frightening looms in front of us. Often, it takes a scary incident like someone wandering out of the house for family members to decide they need to find out what's going on. Whatever the precipitating incident, the important thing is that as a caregiver you made an appointment and agreed to the appropriate tests.

Denial often takes the form of, "Why take my loved one in for testing? I know what it is and there is no cure anyway." But sometimes what looks like dementia isn't, which is why it does matter that you get a diagnosis. Other conditions can mimic dementia—certain thyroid conditions, sleep apnea, vitamin B-12 deficiency. There is also pseudo-dementia, which is a symptom of depression. So, you don't necessarily know what is causing the signs.

In one incident a new person came into the support group and told us that the family doctor had given the parent a diagnosis of Alzheimer's. Something about the description of symptoms, however, aroused my cofacilitator's suspicions. As a neuropsychologist, he obviously had medical knowledge that I didn't have. He asked a number of questions and then suggested that it could be a case of tapeworms that had migrated into the brain (neurocysticercosis). When the parent was seen by a neurologist, it turned out that the symptoms were in fact neurocysticercosis. So, without a thorough examination, and maybe even a second opinion in some cases, you can't know for certain what is wrong with your loved one.

§

If everything else is ruled out and the diagnosis is dementia, I think it's important that the doctor be the one to inform the patient. Most of the time, doctors will go ahead and tell the individual that it is dementia. But sometimes the doctor will inform whichever family member has medical power of attorney and then leave it to that person to pass along the devastating news. Perhaps the physician feels that the news might be better received from a family member. However, everyone has a tendency to blame the messenger. It's better in the long run if the patient is angry at the doctor and not at the family member who will be the caregiver. Breaking the news also puts an enormous amount of pressure on the family member. A couple of people in my support group had been burdened with the task, and it seemed unfair that, with all they were going through, they had to shoulder this responsibility as well.

This situation hits close to home for me. My father was diagnosed with Alzheimer's many months before he was told about it. I actually don't blame the doctor, because I believe this was a result of my mother's instruction. In any event, my understanding is that after my father fell off a horse in 1989 and sustained a head injury that required surgery, there were some suspicious findings when an MRI was done. After that, more attention was given to his brain in his yearly checkups.

I can't recall precisely when the diagnosis was made, but my mother told my brother Ron, who then told me but swore me to secrecy. He made it clear that our father had not been informed. I come from a family in which you almost need Post-it notes on your bathroom mirror to remind you of the latest secret or subterfuge. Anyone with a similar dynamic in their family will relate when I say it's exhausting. Secrets are weighty things; they crush the breath out of you and don't allow you room to evaluate what's really going on. Whenever I hear about families concealing a loved one's diagnosis, I think about the added burden they're putting on an already burdensome situation.

Families are messy. Mine certainly was, and I've now counseled enough people to be able to say with confidence that there are many families in the complicated column. I'm sure my mother felt that she was doing the right thing; I am sure others feel it's right to withhold this vital piece of information, at least for a while. I just don't happen to agree.

Here is the problem: People know when there is something wrong with their brain. They know they are forgetting things; they know the place they are in shouldn't look strange to them, yet it does. If they aren't given a truthful explanation of their symptoms, their fear spreads out in all directions. I believe people deserve the dignity of being fully informed about what's wrong with them. Obviously, it's an individual decision, and some might fervently disagree with me and feel that ignorance is best, that a suitable time for disclosure will make itself known. But I note that if it were any other disease besides dementia, this question wouldn't even come up. I doubt a doctor would pass off a cancer diagnosis to a family member and say, "You tell them." And I doubt that family members would decide to withhold information about a cancer diagnosis.

A common initial diagnosis is Mild Cognitive Impairment, which is generally a prelude to dementia, when the symptoms of memory loss and confusion are noticeable but not terribly bad. I noticed in my support group that many people who received a diagnosis of MCI for their loved ones were not given a complete picture by their doctors. They hadn't been told that in all likelihood things would progress to dementia of some kind, and so they were relieved to hear they had Mild Cognitive Impairment and assumed this was the final diagnosis. While there have been cases of people remaining at that level and not getting worse, it doesn't usually happen like that. When it does, it's often because the individual is elderly and passes away before dementia can set in.

Mild Cognitive Impairment is a warning bell. It means you have to be vigilant in noticing if the symptoms get worse, and then follow up with a complete diagnostic exam to determine what type of dementia your loved one has. The type of dementia is extremely important. When I first began my support group, I was surprised when people came in and asked what the difference was between Alzheimer's and dementia. Or said that their parent had Alzheimer's, but not dementia. I quickly realized that doctors don't always take the time to explain a diagnosis completely or offer context.

By choosing to run Beyond Alzheimer's in a hospital, I learned a lot about how the medical profession works—some of it good, some not. There are many wonderful, compassionate doctors who care about their patients and take time with them. As we have seen in the coronavirus pandemic, there are heroic medical professionals who risk their own health to help those who are ill. I have worked in my support group with doctors who are dedicated and who care deeply about their patients, but sadly there are also doctors and hospital administrators who see medicine as a business and seem to forget that they are dealing with human beings at their most vulnerable stages. I would be remiss if I didn't address some of the attitudes in the medical community toward dementia—an incurable disease that affects mostly the elderly.

After Beyond Alzheimer's had run for five years at UCLA, an administrative change at the highest level made it clear to me that the support group was going to be terminated. I fought to keep it there, but the doctor with the ultimate power wouldn't even meet with me. He finally agreed to a phone call, and during that call he said something I will never forget: "Alzheimer's is the least profitable area of medicine." It's a shockingly callous thing to say, but unfortunately I don't think he's alone in that perception. I made up my mind in that moment to move my group to another hospital before he could shut me down because I was not going to let him have the last word. I moved the group to Saint John's Medical Center and had a much more positive experience with the doctors there, but that cruel comment about the profitability of Alzheimer's has stayed with me and probably always will.

It was glaringly obvious that caregivers and family members should walk into a doctors' office armed with information, in case you get a doctor who does not give you the time and the consideration that you deserve. You might consider getting another doctor if this occurs, or at least seeking out other sources of information.

I mentioned earlier that dementia is a category of disease and Alzheimer's is one type of dementia. There are other types, each with its own peculiarities. Alzheimer's is the most common but is diagnosed only after the other possibilities are ruled out. What type of dementia a person has matters because it tells you what to expect. Every individual is different when it comes to how the disease will manifest. It's said that if you've seen one person with Alzheimer's, you've seen one person with Alzheimer's. But there are some predictable markers and patterns characteristic of each type of dementia. I am not a medical doctor, but since this book focuses primarily on Alzheimer's, I offer a layman's version of the other types of dementia, with added detail about early-onset Alzheimer's and frontotemporal dementia, both of which strike at a young age and don't get as much attention as Alzheimer's.

Vascular Dementia

Vascular dementia is generally the result of a stroke, or a transischemic attack (TIA) when blood flow to the brain is slowed and interrupted. It can also develop over time from other health conditions that affect blood flow to the brain. It typically comes on suddenly and dramatically, but then proceeds in a step-like fashion, which is different from Alzheimer's. During the in-between times, the person can be fairly stable, until another step downward worsens their condition. Vascular dementia is diagnosed with an MRI.

Lewy Body Dementia

Lewy body dementia is a brutal form of dementia. Many might remember that this was what the actor Robin Williams had, although we now know that the diagnosis was not made until an autopsy was conducted after he committed suicide. The documentary *Robin's Wish* details the months of agony and despair Robin and his wife went through as brain scans revealed nothing, yet Robin knew something was terribly wrong. He was feeling himself slip away. Dr. Bruce Miller, a behavioral neurologist who directs the UCSF Dementia Center, and who appears in the film, says that Lewy body dementia "becomes progressively irreversible, unstoppable, and always fatal."[4]

In very simple terms, it's a combination of Parkinson's and dementia, but more complicated. Protein deposits called Lewy bodies attach themselves to the nerve cells in the brain that affect movement, memory, and thinking. Often the first signs are Parkinsonian—tremors, balance issues. Memory does start to go, but it's a roller coaster. Some days might be pretty good, then the next days are literally hell. Hallucinations are typically part of Lewy body dementia; for some reason, the hallucinations are frequently of animals. Auditory hallucinations can also occur. Several people in my support groups had loved ones diagnosed with Lewy body dementia, and the stories were heartbreaking. The hallucinations became terrifying and there was nothing that could be done about them. All that the caregivers could do was endure the screams and, often, hysteria until a moment of respite came and the hallucinations passed.

The diagnosis is a bit more involved and may include blood tests for biomarkers. Cognitive testing is an important part of the diagnosis. Because of the brutality of this disease, it's vital to get an accurate diagnosis, although, as became evident with Robin Williams, this can often be a challenge. Caring for someone with Lewy body dementia is different because of the physical symptoms. A lot more thought has to go into who the caregivers are going to be.

One evening a new person came into the support group and described his parent's condition, which had been diagnosed as Alzheimer's, not by a neurologist but—as is often the case—by the family physician. Aricept had been prescribed in hopes of slowing down the march of the disease. It is in no way a cure, but it's one of the few medications that doctors can offer, so I understand why they offer it. But from what was being said, my cofacilitator and I both didn't think that this individual had Alzheimer's. It sounded, from the symptoms, as though it could be Lewy body dementia, and Aricept is not recommended for that disease. We urged this new group member to get a second opinion. That second examination, by a neurologist, revealed that it was, in fact, Lewy body dementia.

An accurate diagnosis is always important, but with Lewy body dementia it is particularly necessary so that contraindicated medications aren't given to the patient, and so that caregivers can be watchful for the physical, Parkinsonian symptoms that accompany this type of dementia.

Creutzfeldt-Jakob Disease (CJD)

CJD is a fatal degenerative brain disease and is very rare, but because it leads quickly to dementia and has been called Alzheimer's-on-steroids, I include it here. The symptoms, predominantly dementia, behavioral changes, vision loss, and poor coordination, descend in a few months. Patients can even end up in a coma. Death typically occurs within a year. In the six years of running my support group, I never had anyone come in whose loved one had CJD, but outside the group I have met two people whose spouses died from it. They barely had time to emerge from a state of shock after hearing the diagnosis before their spouses died—that's how quickly the disease moved.

Early-Onset Alzheimer's

After a while, I knew the look as soon as I saw it. Someone new would come into the support group full of a grief so deep it was like a bottomless well. Often they would be defensive, as if they were going to challenge anyone's efforts to try to soothe their pain. My instinct would be that their spouse or partner had been diagnosed with early-onset Alzheimer's. I wished that I was wrong, because the stories are so heartbreaking. But I never was.

We expect to lose our parents at some point. That's how life's wheel is supposed to turn. And even though a diagnosis of dementia is devastating, it still exists within the framework of how life is meant to evolve—the passing of an older generation, which allows the next one to step forward in ways they couldn't before. We kneel beside children and explain that grandma or grandpa has a disease that's going to make them act differently, and there is no cure for it. It will keep getting worse. All the while we know we are teaching them one of the most somber and necessary lessons of life—that death comes in many guises, and all we can do is accept it and know that it's part of everyone's cycle.

But how do you explain to a child that a mother or father who is still young, maybe even in their early fifties, has a disease that elderly people usually get? How do you keep children from feeling betrayed by life, by fate, when you feel betrayed and confused? You had plans for the future. There were countries you wanted to visit and chapters of your children's lives that you imagined and discussed late at night in shared whispers. All of that has been taken away.

A man whose wife was diagnosed with early-onset Alzheimer's when she was barely into her fifties told me he worried that their daughter, who was eleven when her mother initially started showing symptoms, would forget what she used to be like and only remember her as splintered by a disease that was making her unrecognizable. I wished I could offer him something that would alleviate the helplessness he felt, but sadly helplessness is part of Alzheimer's, and with early-onset, it's even more pronounced.

A fairly well-known story tells of a large family in Medellín, Colombia, that has for generations been ravaged by a type of early-onset Alzheimer's that almost always claims family members in their mid-forties.[5] It is a sprawling extended family of roughly six thousand people, and their history of early-onset Alzheimer's goes back centuries. They called the disease "La Bobera"[6] which means "the foolishness," and they initially attributed superstitious causes to it.

When they were studied, it was discovered that they had a genetic mutation which, unlike other mutations, was unusually penetrant, so that those who carried it were basically destined to get this type of dementia. In fact, their odds of getting it were about 99 percent. Researchers believe that a Spanish conquistador who traveled to the New World in the sixteenth century had the gene and was the starting point for generations of the disease. Family members who test positive for the gene are being studied for possible treatments and cures. Since it is known in advance that they will get early-onset Alzheimer's, they are valuable sources for research.

This is an unusual genetic mutation. But people who are dealing with early-onset Alzheimer's in their own families often cite this story as evidence that they should be terrified of inheriting the disease and passing it down to their children and grandchildren. I know people who have taken their adolescent children for genetic testing to see if they have any kind of genetic marker that would put them at risk. After all, they reason, there is this story about a family in Colombia.

It's human nature to read stories selectively—we either fixate on what we want to hear or on the things that correspond to our fears. It's clear in all versions of this story about the Medellín family that theirs is a unique genetic mutation, so it really has no bearing on other types of early-onset Alzheimer's. What would be the plan for young teenagers being tested? The APOE gene (apolipoprotein E) has been associated with an elevated risk for Alzheimer's, but only one type (APOE e4) is thought to possibly increase the risk. Everyone has two APOE genes; not everyone has the type that seems to be a risk factor for dementia. And having that gene is not a guarantee that someone will develop the disease. So if those kids tested positive for that particular gene, would they have been told they might get Alzheimer's? That would be an awfully harsh sentence to impose on someone who hadn't even reached adulthood.

The question of why this has happened comes up often with all versions of dementia, but it is even more prevalent when someone young is stricken with a disease we associate with elderly people. We know there is no answer; still, the question lingers, won't let go.

In some instances, if there has been a family history of early-onset Alzheimer's going back through generations, it's possible to blame a genetic link, but the genetics of Alzheimer's is a very murky field. And finding something to blame doesn't lessen the trauma or stop the avalanche of sorrow.

To endure losing a spouse or partner to dementia when they are in the prime of their life is, without a doubt, devastating. But that's all the more reason to attempt what seems impossible—keeping fear in check. It's excruciating to witness a person in the prime of life struggling to remember things, searching for words, ragged with confusion. If it's a person you love and have built a life with, you'll struggle to remember who they once were. You don't want those memories to fade, yet the person who is now in front of you, who doesn't know how to button their shirt, is crowding out those memories. The only way through this is through it. There are no shortcuts, there is no magical formula for transcending the loss. The only lifeline to hold onto is your love for the human being you chose to spend your life with.

Frontotemporal Dementia (FTD)

A nineteen-year-old girl, in her second year of college, goes home for the holidays and watches in horror as her father makes lewd and inappropriate comments to any female within sight. Intermittently he explodes into rage and then sinks into a state of apathy and indifference toward everyone around him. It's painfully clear that he has no empathy for anyone, even his own family. Her mother hadn't wanted to tell her on the phone, especially since the diagnosis is so unexpected and required some time and a lot of testing to complete. She hears her mother say "frontotemporal dementia." But it's the word "dementia" that slams into her. Her father is in his fifties. How could this be real?

Her father will never see her graduate from college, never walk her down the aisle when she gets married, never meet his grand-children. Entire chapters of the future she thought they would share have vanished with the diagnosis of frontotemporal dementia.

A woman with three very young children, pregnant with her fourth child, asks her husband to watch the kids while she runs some errands. When she returns, she finds two of the kids playing out-side, unsupervised, next to a busy road. Her husband is inside the house watching television, oblivious and uncaring. Over the next few months his apathy increases. He doesn't seem to care about any of them. He begins eating voraciously, not out of hunger, but out of some mysterious compulsion that drives him to put almost any-thing in his mouth. She locks up the food, but he goes to the store and buys more. She cuts up his credit cards, and he goes to the store and steals food. He is fired from his job for making lewd comments to a coworker.

This second story about frontotemporal dementia was featured in a *60 Minutes* segment entitled "The Cruelest Disease You Have Never Heard Of."[7] The segment looked into the lives of Amy and Mark Johnson and the nightmare of a young woman whose husband is not even remotely the man she fell in love with and has to be put into a facility. There he eats constantly, puts on a hundred pounds, and wants his wife and children to leave a few minutes after they arrive for a visit. He is in his early forties. The facility costs $13,000 a month; their life savings is disappearing. One can't say that her hope is disappearing, because she hasn't had any.

Dr. Bruce Miller, who has done extensive work with FTD, participated in the *60 Minutes* piece. He said about the disease, "It attacks people at the very soul of their humanity."[8]

It attacks the entire family, too, which of course is true about any form of dementia. But because FTD strikes a person at a relatively young age, it forces small children to grow up too quickly and learn about the unfairness of life in the tender years when they still believe in Santa Claus.

⁂

THERE ARE THREE VARIANTS of FTD, behavioral and two language forms—non-fluent aphasia and semantic. The behavioral variant is the most common. As with Amy and Mark Johnson, very young children may watch helplessly as a parent initially loses interest in them and seemingly in life itself, then see that parent's behavior become explosive, out of place, and embarrassing. For example, people stricken with behavioral dementia might walk over to another table in a restaurant and take a stranger's food, or shoplift. Their interactions with others, even passersby, can be terribly inappropriate.

In non-fluent aphasia, the variant that affects speech and language, the left side of the frontal lobe, responsible for naming objects and pronouncing words, is affected. So, the person develops difficulty in communicating as well as reading and writing. In the semantic variant, a subtype that predominantly involves the temporal lobes, there is loss of knowledge of words.

Unlike in Alzheimer's, memory is not really affected in the initial stages of frontotemporal dementia. At least in the early stages of Alzheimer's, people have an awareness of what they are losing, of what is falling apart in them. That's not the case with FTD. With this dementia, people don't realize how they are behaving.

When I started Beyond Alzheimer's, I knew about FTD but had never encountered anyone who was going through it with a loved one. The first time someone came into the support group and began describing the behavior, I educated myself about the disease, but I felt an inescapable sense of futility. As much as I believe, in all circumstances, that one's soul can't be ill, it felt almost trivial to say that to someone whose parent or partner was unraveling before their eyes. I had to remind myself that being listened to is important, and perhaps the person in front of me who was describing impossible situations of rage and unpredictability was being helped simply by having a group of people willingly and generously listening to them. I'm not implying that we didn't try to offer suggestions—we did—but FTD presents a completely different set of challenges than those that come with Alzheimer's.

More often than not, getting an accurate diagnosis is problematic. Because FTD strikes people who are young, the first suspicions are that the individual might have a psychiatric personality disorder. Doctors don't initially consider dementia. It can be time-consuming to get the right diagnosis; it can even take years. In some cases people with undiagnosed FTD may make irresponsible financial decisions that can't be reversed; some are arrested for antisocial behavior that crosses a line and violates the law. The home environment turns nightmarish. Even the aphasia of verbal FTD upends life as usual. The person can't find the words he or she needs, can't form sentences. Communication becomes a guessing game for the caregiver. Getting an accurate diagnosis as quickly and early as possible is vitally important.

Once the diagnosis is made, especially with the behavioral variant, it's very difficult to keep the person at home. But placing them in a facility means putting a young, disturbed person, who is acting inappropriately most of the time, in the company of elderly residents who are suffering from more common forms of dementia. The story of Amy and Mark Johnson is not uncommon. People with FTD may be asked to leave facilities.

As a facilitator of a support group, I felt helpless listening to a story involving FTD that was spilling out in front of me. But that, of course, was a fraction of what the group member telling the story felt. There are surprises and unexpected changes in every form of dementia. With FTD, though, the surprises are like a hundred-year storm that just moved in—everything suddenly changes. I have searched online and in consultation with doctors for something helpful I could pass along to people. Here are some behavioral suggestions.

One is the importance of identifying triggers. It may take a lot of detective work, especially if the person has the verbal variant of FTD and can't communicate. But try reducing noise, lessening clutter, and simplifying social interactions. Someone with any kind of dementia, but particularly FTD, can easily be upset by an excess of noise. Noise is annoying to most of us, but we have the ability to reason and think it through. We can tell ourselves that it's temporary, or we can figure out someplace to go while the noise is going on. Someone with FTD doesn't have that ability. If it's a situation out of your control—construction next door, for example—the caregiver might take the person for a walk someplace where it's quiet.

Clutter may be a trigger because an overly cluttered environment may feel out of one's control and risky: something could fall, or there might be unknown things lurking behind those piles of stuff. So creating organized surroundings may be a help.

Simplifying social interactions is good advice for any kind of dementia. Questions are never a good idea—they put pressure on individuals with dementia who feel that they should answer but don't know how. With FTD, the reactions are probably going to be much more extreme.

Other specific suggestions for dealing with some of the out-of-control behavior that is characteristic of FTD include, for the inappropriate sexual advances and the compulsion to touch strangers, often inappropriately, that are typical, giving the person a squeeze ball, so that his or her hands are occupied, or providing a large stuffed animal for them to hold. I don't have any personal knowledge that these methods work, but with a disease as extreme as frontotemporal dementia, it's a good idea to give all reasonable suggestions a try.

There is encouraging evidence regarding the benefits of exercise for people who have FTD. Kaitlin Casaletto, PhD, assistant professor of neurology at UCSF Memory and Aging Center, studied a group of people who had been diagnosed with FTD. She found that among the participants who had more active lifestyles, who did some form of exercise, even if it was just brisk walking, functional decline was roughly 55 percent slower. This doesn't mean that the disease itself was reversed; it means that the symptoms were reduced. This could be extremely important for families who are dealing with the behavioral variant of FTD, who never know what to expect as symptoms. It could also lead to some form of treatment to lessen the symptoms as studies continue in an effort to determine exactly what is happening in the brain.[9]

The unique torment of FTD is that those who have it, unlike those with Alzheimer's, become almost unrecognizable. Their apathy, lack of empathy, outbursts, and out-of-control behavior around other people bear no resemblance to the person friends and family once knew. It causes a complicated form of grief for the loved ones and caregivers. It shreds their patience and undermines their emotional stability. If someone is tempted to feel the universe has turned against them, this disease can easily bring on that despair.

Alzheimer's

If Alzheimer's is the diagnosis, commonly prescribed medications such as Aricept may slow down the symptoms. Exelon, Namenda, and Razadyne are also frequently used. They all have possible side effects, so those should be weighed. But consider this before deciding to put a loved one on any of these medications: The early stages of Alzheimer's are the most difficult in the sense that those who have been diagnosed know they are losing cognitive thought. They know their memory is failing. They have a palpable sense of what is being taken from them. I can only imagine the fear that rises up in them every day. I used to see it in my father's eyes—this man who was never afraid of anything. One day he stood in the middle of the living room and said, "I don't know where I am." Fear was coiled tightly in his eyes. It seems to me that some thought should be given to the idea of slowing down the disease at the earlier, more traumatic stages. Is that really where you want your loved one to linger? The uniqueness of Alzheimer's is that, ironically, things get a bit easier—in some ways—as the disease worsens.

It's obviously an individual choice when it comes to medication, and there is no right or wrong here. I just ask you to look at it from all angles. It's obviously tempting to try and slow down an encroaching disease for which there is no cure. But sometimes, with medications, we slow it down at the most difficult stage. I know that with my father there was some relief when he moved beyond knowing that his memory was being stolen from him, when he stopped grasping for recollections, for pieces of his life that were no longer there. He had gotten worse, but, in a strange twist, he was more settled, more serene in that empty landscape.

"We have to go into the despair and go beyond it, by working and doing for somebody else, by using it for something else."

—Elie Wiesel

CHAPTER 2

Taking Away the Car Keys, Opening the Door to an Outside Caregiver

There is so much to think about when dementia is suddenly a reality: it can feel like an avalanche of questions has tumbled down on you. When should I get help for my loved one? Should I still allow them to drive? What about finances? Can they still pay their bills properly? Can they still go out to restaurants and movies? Should I get help in the house now or wait for a while? What if they won't allow someone else to come in?

The best thing I can tell you is that you have time. You don't have to answer every question that arises right now. In fact, there will come a point down the line when time seems to move so slowly it almost becomes the enemy. But that's later. At the beginning, you do need to acknowledge that all the questions I mentioned, and more, will have to be dealt with eventually. But you can start with the most immediate ones. Like driving and caregiving.

In California, when a doctor makes a diagnosis of any type of dementia, he or she is legally mandated to report that to the Department of Motor Vehicles. This is not the case in every state; only 12 percent of the states have such a law. In those states, the DMV then contacts the individual, who must come in for a driver's test, and in many cases, will issue a temporary license, generally for six months. The DMV is typically very slow, so waiting for a summons may not be the best idea. It might be better to be proactive: set up an appointment yourself. A person with Alzheimer's, or any kind of dementia, can rally themselves to pass the tests they're taking. Sometimes someone who really should not be driving diligently studies the written material, as if studying for a college exam, and passes the test. But the fact that someone passes the tests, even the actual driving test, doesn't mean they should be behind the wheel. If your loved one is showing any signs of impaired judgment (which they must be or you wouldn't have had them diagnosed), you're going to have to figure out how to get the car keys away from them. It's usually one of the more dramatic episodes in the world of Alzheimer's, although I do know of a few people whose loved ones readily gave up driving.

A good rule to follow is one that's successfully used with children: don't take something away without offering a replacement. Explain that it's not safe for them to drive the car anymore, but you're going to set them up with a ride-sharing service like Uber or Lyft. Or you're going to hire someone part time, like a college student, to drive them around. If you're already at the point of getting a caregiver to come in, even for a few hours, make sure it's someone who drives.

There might still be high drama around this. Think about it—when you first got your driver's license, it was a huge deal. You were independent, you could go where you wanted when you wanted.

It was one of the best days of your life. So, losing that independence becomes one of the worst. It cuts deep.

I'm pretty sure I've heard every rationalization imaginable for not taking the car away from a loved one: They only drive a short distance. They never go on the freeway. They drive slowly. I've ridden with them and nothing happened. They seemed to be paying attention. They stopped for the cyclist who went through the stop sign.

A person with dementia does not have the same awareness of their surroundings as someone without the disease. The synapses in their brains are not working as they should. Driving requires split-second reactions; if those reactions don't occur, or occur too late, lives can be lost. I understand the reluctance to confront a loved one about this—it's hard. But it will be far worse if a child on a bicycle is killed, or a pedestrian is hit.

I've heard incredibly creative methods for getting the car away from someone who should no longer be driving it. One person got advice from a mechanic and disabled the car, then had it towed away, claiming the "repair" was taking a very long time, and after months passed their parent forgot about it. Another person paid a neighbor to drive the car away, then said it was stolen and it wasn't feasible financially to get another car. Eventually the person with Alzheimer's does forget. Maybe not immediately, and definitely not as quickly as you'd like them to, but they do forget.

❧

ON JULY 16, 2003, an eighty-six-year-old man named George Weller drove his 1992 Buick LeSabre through the streets of Santa Monica, California, heading toward the weekly Farmer's Market.[10] It was a little before two in the afternoon, and the market was packed with people. He ploughed through a road closure sign and several wooden sawhorses, straight into the crowd of people, accelerating as he went. With bodies bouncing off the hood of his car, he went between forty and sixty miles an hour for two and a half blocks. His car didn't stop until it hit a ditch. Two bodies were splayed on the hood of his car and a woman was trapped beneath the car.

Weller got out of the car with the same dazed look he reportedly had while he was speeding down the street. Amid blood and bodies, collapsed fruit stands, and screaming bystanders, he stepped out into sunshine, looked around and asked, "How many people did I hit?"

He killed ten people and injured sixty-three.

He claimed to have hit the gas instead of the brake, and that became his lawyer's defense when he was charged with vehicular manslaughter. It didn't work. George Weller, who either lacked remorse or didn't understand what he'd done, was charged with ten counts of vehicular manslaughter.

He had not been diagnosed with dementia, although the possibility that he might in fact have had dementia was brought up. It was discovered that he had been involved in another accident ten years earlier, when he again drove his car aimlessly, having no idea what he was doing or what he had done once he stopped. Fortunately, no one was injured or killed then, but it was clear that someone should have intervened and taken his car away from him years before that horrible summer day.

I cite this story frequently when people tell me it's just too difficult to get the car keys away from their parent or spouse. I use the story for a very specific reason—to scare the hell out of them. This is how bad it can get. The carnage of that day took less than a minute. Ten people, including a baby, died. Sixty-three others were seriously injured. Lawsuits for millions of dollars were filed.

In all likelihood, your loved one is not going to want to hand over the car keys. But, unfortunately, they have been diagnosed with a disease that makes driving a very dangerous activity. The simple truth is, they don't get a vote in this matter.

❧

THE OTHER AREA OF contention that comes up pretty quickly is the idea of hiring an outside caregiver, even for a few days a week. It's not only the person with dementia who might resist this: some family members don't like the idea of a "stranger" coming in, or feel as if they can do the job themselves.

If your elderly parent has been diagnosed with Alzheimer's and lives alone, there are serious risks in them continuing to be alone. Even in the early stages, it only takes one instance of leaving the stove on and walking away to burn the house down. What if they walk out the door, wander off, and forget where they are? What if they let a stranger into the house, mistakenly believing that they know the person? Or go to sleep at night with the front door wide open?

You're probably going to have a difficult time convincing someone who has been accustomed to living alone to suddenly have a caregiver loitering around. And financially it may be a burden. You can start gradually, though, hiring someone for a few hours here and there. If there are no other medical issues, if a hired caregiver is primarily there for companionship and to monitor things, the cost is generally not prohibitive. Alternatively, during the daytime there are senior day care centers, which often provide transportation. These centers, at least the reputable ones, offer art classes, music, even dancing. It's a way to keep a parent stimulated and around other people so they don't sink into isolation. Depression is quite common in the early stages of dementia because the person is aware of what is slipping away from them. Activity and socialization, which day care centers provide, can make a huge difference.

In the early stages it generally isn't necessary to have someone with a nursing degree, so the cost is less. Of course, for some families any expenditure for outside caregiving is a burden. A growing number face financial devastation because one member has been diagnosed with some form of dementia. Even a "companion" caregiver who might only charge twenty dollars an hour is a stretch, because it adds up. Cost was not a problem my parents had to deal with, but I am acutely aware of the financial strain this disease puts on too many families. At the risk of getting political, I think it is shameful that in America we have not fixed our health care system so that no family has to lose everything when a terminal diagnosis is handed down and outside care is needed. At some point, America is going to have to fix what is broken—a health care system that doesn't take care of people in need.

A man who was a regular in my support group when it first started had a great suggestion. He told people to thoroughly read their life insurance and health insurance policies because sometimes, in the fine print, there are allowances for a certain number of hours of outside care. These aren't things we generally notice when we sign up, because who actually reads every page of an insurance policy? If you combine what each policy allows, you might find that it enables you to have someone come in for a few hours several days a week.

OFTEN PEOPLE DECIDE THAT the best solution for dealing with a parent who has Alzheimer's is to have that parent move in with a son or daughter. In cases where the relationship has been strong, the adult child is motivated by love and a willingness to make sacrifices. But in other scenarios, a son or daughter who has a troubled history with the parent might think they can finally find love and harmony in these last stages of life—the love and harmony that were never there before. No matter what the family history is, here is the problem: caregiving is a full-time job. It leaves little room for the emotions that can rise up in a son or daughter, emotions that ask to be acknowledged and explored. If you had a close, loving relationship with the loved one who is now ill, the best thing you can do for both of you is to nurture that. You can't do that if you are taking on the role of hands-on caregiver, making yourself responsible for all their physical needs. You can't play both roles. If hiring an outside caregiver is not possible because of financial constraints, you need to carve out some time—literally schedule it—when you can step down from being the caregiver and simply be the daughter, the son, the spouse, the partner, and grieve for the person you are losing. Reserve some time each day to sit alone and cry, or daydream, or just be alone. Make it a priority. Ask a friend or a family member to sit with the person who is ill if need be, but give yourself that time.

A frequent comment when it comes to a parent is, "Well, they took care of me when I was a child, so it seems right that I take care of them now." To be blunt, it's not the same thing. Children grow out of diapers and high chairs and the need to be fed and bathed. An adult with dementia does not; in fact, the movement goes the other way. That adult will get worse and will need trained people to help. This is not a virus, or recovery from surgery; this is a progressive, debilitating disease that worsens according to its own timetable.

Early on in writer Marianne Williamson's career she did a lot of work with AIDS patients, including support groups. One of the things she said about the seriousness of the disease and all the challenges that arise from it was, "We're not talking about the flu here." I would say the same about Alzheimer's. Everything needs to be reevaluated—your agendas, your ideas about how things "should" be, your personal history. We all like to think we are in control of our future, but dealing with dementia is like being dropped into a foreign country. You're going to have to learn new ways, and a new language.

Leaving the hands-on caregiving to someone else doesn't mean that you're not a caregiver. You're providing the emotional care that no one else can. Caregiving has many facets—companionship, feeding, bathing, dressing, keeping watch, but it also includes emotional sustenance and the reinforcement of the bond of love that disease can't take away. You owe it to yourself, and to your loved one, to give the emotional facet of caregiving the reverence it deserves.

If your relationship with your parent was difficult and challenging throughout your life, Alzheimer's is not going to suddenly transform it into something sweet and loving. But if you give yourself the space and the time to explore this new chapter, if you loosen your grip on the past, you might figure out how to see that parent differently, through more forgiving eyes. That won't happen if you are exhausted from getting them dressed, fixing them meals, and everything else that goes into being a full-time caregiver. You simply will not have the time or energy for your own emotional journey.

We weren't trained to be full-time caregivers for people with dementia. It's a unique skill set. But there are people who have been trained in this vocation, and including them in your life—in your parent's life—will allow you to let go of your mother or father in the ways that you need to as the disease steals them away.

With the coronavirus pandemic, an increasing number of people have removed their loved ones from facilities because of concern they will contract the virus. They have no option but to bring their relative into their home. If you're a caregiver in this situation, it's essential also to make caring for yourself a priority. Take time to nurture yourself—time away from your home, away from your loved one. Find someone to sit with them for an hour or two, then drive to the beach, go on a hike, visit a friend. But monitor where your thoughts are: if they are still in your house, if you're worrying about what might be happening or what could go wrong, you're not taking a break—you're just changing the scenery.

No matter your circumstances in terms of caregiving, you need to know the pitfalls and how best to keep yourself sane and healthy. There is an added emotional weight to caring for a loved one with dementia, beyond just the physical toll. This is especially true if you are taking on the entire burden yourself. If you can't change the external reality, you can still strengthen yourself emotionally by understanding all aspects of your situation—the internal as well as the external. Stress has landed many caregivers in the hospital, so make caring for yourself a priority.

If you have never taken up meditation before, this is a good time to start. Studies have shown the mental benefits of meditating even just twenty minutes a day, among them a decrease in cortisol, the stress hormone.[11] Keep in mind that in the world of dementia, the caregiver is the one feeling stress, not the patient. Someone with dementia who gets upset or tense will get over it in a short time. You, the caregiver, will not. So, cultivate tools and methods to alleviate the stress and anxiety that will always be clawing at you.

℘

WHEN YOUR PARENTS ARE together and one of them is diagnosed with dementia, you have to deal with the feelings of both—the one who has been diagnosed and is frightened, even angry, and the one who is trying to absorb what this means for their lives going forward. Most of the time, the healthy one will want to care for their spouse, and want to convince themselves that they can handle the job. Let that play out for a while but choose some moments to introduce the idea of hiring a part-time caregiver to help. Wait until it seems this suggestion might be received and seriously considered, then gently bring it up.

Our parents had a life with each other before we came along, and they have a relationship with each other separate from their role as our parents. They need to figure out this part of the journey for themselves. Ultimately, it's not going to be sustainable for an elderly parent, with his or her own health issues, to be caring for a spouse who has Alzheimer's. But changes will go more smoothly if you give both parents some space to adjust to their new reality, all the while keeping a watchful eye on them. There probably will come a time when you have to intervene and insist that a hired caretaker be brought in, but giving your parents a little time to adjust to what fate has handed them will make it a smoother road. If you're lucky, they will figure out on their own that they need help.

My family was in a unique situation, given that my father still had Secret Service protection. Thus there were always people to drive him around, and no risk of him wandering off the property and ending up miles away. In the earliest stages he went into the office for a few hours each day. My mother figured out that maintaining the familiar structure of my father's days was important. Perhaps it was instinct, or just her own need to hold onto the way things had been. Whatever it was, it worked. He relied on getting dressed in his suit and heading to the office just as he had done for years, and the predictability of it seemed to ground him. When his symptoms got worse and going to the office started to become unfeasible, my mother hired someone to help my father through the day at home. There were no medical issues yet, so it was simply for companionship and protection, to ensure that he wouldn't do something risky.

Losing your spouse or partner to dementia is, in so many ways, a different kind of wound. This is your other half, your lover, the person you wanted to grow old with—only not like this. As far as caregiving goes, it's especially important for someone losing their other half to have the room to absorb how enormous the loss is, to not get pulled away from that reality by the burden of hands-on caregiving. You can't play both roles. If possible, let someone who is trained to care for dementia patients deal with the day-to-day duties, so you can deal with the challenge of saying goodbye in stages, which is what Alzheimer's brings you to.

❧

A QUESTION THAT HOVERS in the background almost from the beginning is, "Who is my loved one going to be now, with this disease?"

The answer is pretty simple and may or may not be what you want to hear. With the exception of frontotemporal dementia, the person with dementia, particularly Alzheimer's, is going to be who they always were underneath the social niceties and protective layers that we all develop in life. So if at their core they were kind and gentle individuals, that's what will remain. If they were complaining and mean-spirited, hang on, because it's going to get worse. A woman I know, whose mother had Alzheimer's, talked about violent episodes in which her mother threw things, screamed at the top of her lungs, was mean to caregivers. I had crossed paths with her mother several times many years earlier, long before the diagnosis of Alzheimer's, and let's just say I was never surprised by any of these reports.

Alzheimer's erodes the filters that every person has. What is left after that erosion is the essential self. My father, for example, was a very kind-hearted man, and he remained so throughout the ten years of Alzheimer's. It doesn't mean there weren't times of upset and even bursts of anger—there were. But who he was at his core remained intact.

People have said to me that they never saw a sweet side of their mother, or a hostile, demanding side of their father before Alzheimer's, so the disease must have created these characteristics; it must have transformed them into someone else. Each time, as we talked more and they shuffled through memories, it became clear that these qualities were there, and peeked out sometimes. One man swore to me that his father only became a racist when he was overtaken by Alzheimer's. Dementia does not cause racism. His father apparently did a good job of concealing his prejudice throughout much of his life, but it was in there. It reminds me of a palimpsest—a painting created over other paintings. With time, the layers start to fade and what's underneath becomes visible, until what you finally see is the original painting.

It's a bit of a life lesson, if you think about it. We all might examine who we are beneath the face we present to the world. One way or another, people usually are revealed in time, even if disease doesn't enter the picture. If we know we have anger and are judgmental, but we cover these feelings up throughout our lives, they won't stay covered up forever.

One day, an elderly woman behind the wheel of a badly dented car almost clipped me at an intersection as she was making a left turn. I honked to alert her that she was coming within inches of me; she scrunched up her face and stuck out her tongue. I wondered about her afterward—if when she was a younger woman, that impulse was there but she never acted on it.

It can be extremely difficult to be around someone with dementia who is unpleasant and mean a lot of the time. Even the most patient and good-natured people will ultimately get annoyed. The way to get respite from that annoyance is to change your perspective. Think about the fact that people with dementia can no longer change who they are; they don't have the tools. Time and disease have taken away that option. How sad to leave this world rooted in the unhealthy choices of anger and meanness.

Looking at it from that angle may not take away all your frustration, but it will probably add sympathy to the mix. And that's a softer place to be. Sympathy and compassion are always reliable antidotes. (It's also okay to leave the room for a bit to clear your head.)

❧

ALZHEIMER'S IS A DISEASE with a big reach—to some degree, it consumes everyone who is around it, even family members who try to stay away, who fool themselves into thinking that geographical distance will lessen the anguish. Often people in my support group complained that their siblings took no responsibility; in fact, they stayed as far away as they could from the parent who had Alzheimer's. "They won't help at all!" was a cry I heard frequently from the caregiver. I usually responded, "Well, that's why God put you there." The truth is that the family members who stay away are cutting themselves off from the profound lessons that this disease can teach. They are not allowing themselves whatever closure they might obtain in their relationship with their parent.

I once went on a date with a man who told me proudly that he was avoiding his father, who had been diagnosed with Alzheimer's, because of their tumultuous relationship. He said he was finally free of his father's abuse and staying away proved that. He said this after ordering his third vodka. I kept my mouth shut, but it was clear to me that this man wasn't free of anything.

Those of us who do stay, who do show up, tend to think that we have to take huge, heroic steps to deal with the situation. But that's not true. Small moments, gestures that might seem insignificant, can make a big difference to someone whose memory is abandoning them. That person may not be able to navigate his or her way through the day without help, but can still recognize kindness and will respond to connection. These are some of the feelings that Alzheimer's cannot extinguish; it helps to remember that.

"There is no such thing as a great deed. Only small deeds done with great love."　　　　　　　　　—MOTHER TERESA

CHAPTER 3

Grief Arrives Early

We tend to think of grief as something we have to deal with after a loved one dies. Before that, as disease ravages the person we love, we refer to our sorrow, our despair, the waves of tears that come at odd times. But we don't usually mention grief. We consider the weightiness of grief as something that awaits us at the end, after death. Alzheimer's, though, is a death before dying. So grief needs to be embraced early on. You will watch as the person you know so well fades from view. Alzheimer's piracy is unpredictable and unrelenting. The disease is in control; it will steal what it chooses when it chooses and there is nothing you can do to stop it.

When I sat with my father, I anchored myself in the faith that his soul was unencumbered by dementia. I imagined a clear, calm lake far beneath the choppy waters of Alzheimer's. I felt I had entered a different reality, a sort of suspended state where I could look at the disease from enough of a distance that, no matter what was going on physically, his spirit still whispered to me. Those visits had a serenity to them, despite my sorrow. I would often drive away from my parents' house and have to pull over to the side of the road to sit in my car and cry. This is my reality now, I told myself. I'm straddling two worlds—the spiritual realm of faith in the soul's endurance, its imperviousness to disease, and the physical realm of loss, helplessness, and sorrow beyond measure.

Grief constantly asks us to acknowledge it. Most of us want to avoid it, for the obvious reason that it hurts. And Alzheimer's offers ample opportunities for avoidance. You can keep yourself so busy with caregiving duties that you have no time to grieve or even think about grief. This is one of the reasons people plunge into hands-on caregiving. Intuitively, they know they won't have time to wrestle with the enormity of their loss. And somewhere in all that busyness is the idea that maybe, if they just ignore grief long enough, it will go away and they'll never have to deal with it.

But it doesn't work like that. Grief is not biodegradable. You can't send it out to the farthest field and wait for it to decompose. You might be able to avoid it for months, even years. But eventually it will come find you. When that happens, it usually stops you in your tracks with an illness, or an accident—something that will leave you no choice but to sink into the heartbreak you've been avoiding.

Many years ago I knew a woman whose husband had died of cancer. He was at home for the last stages of the disease, after it was determined that there was nothing more the doctors could do. She took on the task of primary caregiver, allowing little or no help in the house. It wasn't because of financial limitations, it was simply a choice she made. A couple of months after he died, she suddenly became agoraphobic—she couldn't leave her house. She would open the door and a panic attack would slam her back in. She was wise enough to quickly figure out what it was. She told me that she had kept herself so busy caring for her husband, she took no time to grieve. When she was suddenly unable to leave her house, grief was all she had. She had little choice but to sit there and surrender to it. By the time I met her, she was fine—no more agoraphobia.

WE GRIEVE BECAUSE we have loved. The pain we feel when someone is leaving this world is the pain of a heart that opened itself, was willing to be vulnerable. If you never loved, you would never grieve. But that would be an awful way to go through life. I found myself being grateful for the slow pace of grief that comes with a disease like Alzheimer's. I was grateful that I had time with the stages of loss, with grief's different twists and turns. At nineteen, I lost a close friend very suddenly in a hiking accident. I remember the paralysis of shock, and how it took time to even begin mourning his death. I felt ill equipped to handle both the initial paralysis and the flood of emotions that came after.

As a child, I mourned the deaths of beloved pets. My father consoled me, talked about the beautiful times we'd had with them, and how those times would always be with me. We were always rescuing dogs who had been abandoned near our ranch, so another dog would be brought into our home shortly after an older pet died. My father believed strongly that even though you're grieving, your heart needs to love, and filling the emptiness left by a pet's passing was important. He was brilliant in teaching a child about moving through the sorrow that death brings into life, at least where it concerned animals.

But when my paternal grandmother died, I had to hide my sadness. I wasn't supposed to know. I think my parents believed they were protecting me, but at ten years old I had become adept at eavesdropping and had heard through a closed door that Nelle had passed away. She had been put into a facility when she began showing signs of dementia, and the last time I saw her was when my parents took me for a visit. She was in a narrow bed in a room with about ten other beds. The walls were pea-soup green and the smell of urine hung in the air. It was 1962 and there were very few options for placing elderly people who couldn't live on their own and could no longer care for themselves. I can still picture that room, I can still hear nurses padding across the hard linoleum floor, and I can still see my grandmother's wide, empty eyes. Eventually, my parents told me she had died, and I have a memory of saying, "I know," but I'm not sure if I actually did say that. Grief had suddenly become confusing to me. Why, when one of our family pets died, could we talk about it and share our feelings, but when my grandmother died it was kept hidden from me? To this day, I don't know if there was a service for my grandmother.

As difficult as it may be to shepherd a child through the grieving process, it's profoundly important. Those memories stay with us throughout our life. Our earliest lessons about sorrow and loss help form the foundation of who we are. I vividly remember the loneliness of knowing my grandmother had died but having to keep it to myself. I remember it as a physical pain deep inside my ribcage. And I remember the awful weight of questions—why wouldn't my parents talk to me about it? Was it daytime or night when she died? Was she alone? I still don't know the answers and I never will.

Recently I lost a friend of thirty-five years to a sudden heart attack. I got the news in the evening, and I felt the forces of denial and shock moving into me. I couldn't cry. My mind knew it was true—he was gone—but my heart couldn't absorb it yet. I couldn't fathom the world without him in it. The next day, all I wanted to do was cry. I knew, from the moment I got the news, that I had to let grief move at its own pace. As familiar as grief becomes in our lives, each occurrence seems unique. When this friend died, I felt completely unprepared for the ravages of my emotions. Each time I experience loss, part of me watches the process as if I need to memorize it for the next time, yet I know that next time will have its own imprint and will not resemble anything that came before.

⁊⊚

MY SUPPORT GROUP MET one night shortly after the Orlando nightclub shooting. I remember looking around at the group members who were going through the long goodbye of dementia. It occurred to me that those who lose a loved one in this slow passage might reflect on the gift of time that has been given them. The family and friends of people who are murdered brutally in mass shootings never get to say goodbye, never get to sit beside that person and talk about the life they shared together. They never get a chance to reflect on death as it moves slowly toward them. For them, death comes in a blinding flash of gunfire. In an instant their sons, daughters, husbands, wives, friends are gone. And the victims of such shootings spent their last moments on earth staring into the heart of darkness. Evil defined the end of their lives. That's profoundly different from the experience of being cared for, either at home or in a facility, where they will likely die between soft sheets, surrounded by people who care about them.

For those of us who lose someone to dementia, the one thing we have in abundance is time. The person who is ill also has time. Many things might be going on inside them that they aren't able to communicate, so they might be benefiting from that time in ways we will never know. It's a blessing to be able to say goodbye in stages. In the midst of grieving, it's important to remember that death comes in many ways. And a long goodbye is actually one of the gentler ways. The pain is deep, the sorrow is vast, but it's important to widen our view and consider the losses suffered by others.

❧

ELISABETH KÜBLER ROSS WROTE about five stages of grief, and they are very real: denial, anger, bargaining, sorrow, and acceptance.[12] These don't necessarily unfold in a linear manner, though. Grief is a messy process. You can be deep in sorrow and suddenly stumble into denial. Or you can emerge into a clearing that you know is acceptance, only to find yourself slipping back into anger over the unfairness of the disease. As much as it can feel like Mr. Toad's Wild Ride, giving in to whatever stage of grief you're in is a healthier choice than trying to fight it.

When I was younger, I used to follow my father out into the ocean to bodysurf. He was fearless, heading out to meet huge waves, turning his back and swimming hard to catch the wave at just the right point so he could ride it to shore. He taught me everything I know about the sea, about tides and currents and waves. He taught me that if a wave is about to break on you, dive down deep to where the water is still and wait until it passes over you. He taught me that if you're caught in a current that's pulling you out, you're going to be in more trouble if you fight against it. You'll get exhausted, and the current will win. A better choice is to let yourself be carried for a while and wait until you feel it shift or weaken. Then you'll have the strength to swim back. His lessons about the ocean always seemed to translate to lessons about life. I thought of them often throughout his illness.

There is something lonely and majestic in a swimmer cutting through the water, trailing bubbles and breaking the surface with a clean line of strokes. One of the ways I could always engage my father, even deep into the disease, was to talk about water—either the ocean or the river in the town where he grew up. Long after he had forgotten that he once commanded the world stage, long after he no longer knew he'd been president of the United States, he remembered the river. In the deeply rooted memories that Alzheimer's couldn't kill, he was plunging happily into deep waters, confident that he could master the currents. His eyes would light up when I began reciting to him the stories he had once told me—the icy-white afternoons skating on the river that was "wide as the town and twice as long," and the long days of summer, diving into cool water.

"The river is deceptive," my father used to tell me. "On the surface it looks calm, but underneath there are strong currents." The stories and images that marked my childhood became my sustenance in adulthood, in the seasons of his leaving. I dreamt one night that I was standing on the banks of a river. I was all alone, and I knew I had to cross. I was shivering as I stepped into the water, and then the currents started pulling me. I swam hard but felt at some spots that the currents were too strong for me, and I might drown. I remember the sky in my dream—it looked like early evening, and I was scared that night would move in before I got to the other side. Then I suddenly felt hands pulling me and I glided smoothly through the water to the other side. I stood on the riverbank and looked back across the water; I saw a small shape in the distance, and in the dream I knew it was me—another me, before I crossed the river to the other side.

It was one of those dreams that never fade. It's vivid to this day. I decided to tell my father about it. He was still in the early stages of Alzheimer's, still going to the office for a few hours during the week. At home, he had started to regularly scoop fallen magnolia blossoms out of the pool. Since he had been forbidden to swim, I think it was a way to stay close to the water, and since he clearly enjoyed it, the Secret Service agents used to gather magnolia blossoms and throw them into the pool so he would have more to scoop out.

That's where I found him late on a Sunday morning, sunlight slicing through the trees, the pool scooper rippling the water. I described my dream to him, told him how invisible hands had guided me across the river. I didn't really expect him to say anything, but when I was done, he said, "You gotta keep swimming." I have no idea what meaning lay behind those words, but it's an awfully good description of how to handle grief. Keep swimming.

Michelangelo said that when he looked at a block of marble, he believed the shape that wanted to be born from it already existed. David, the Pietà, Moses were already there. His job as sculptor was simply to remove the excess marble and reveal the shape hidden within the stone. That's how life is supposed to work. Our loves, our joys, our sorrows, and our losses are meant to reveal us—by chipping away at everything that conceals who we are capable of being so we can emerge as the people we were created to be. It just sometimes hurts along the way.

"There is a sacredness in tears. They are not the mark of weakness, but of power. They speak more eloquently than ten thousand tongues. They are messengers of overwhelming grief and unspeakable love."   —Washington Irving

THE EARLY STAGES

CHAPTER 4

Where Is the Person I Knew?

The human brain is full of surprises. There were occasions in my support group when someone would say that their parent or spouse had suddenly regained some lucidity. They almost appeared to be recovering, which is of course impossible. A week later the loved one would be back to where they were before. There is no explaining this, and it can make defining the stages of Alzheimer's tricky at times.

In the nineties, when my father was diagnosed, the available information about Alzheimer's (and there wasn't much) enumerated stages of the disease, as if there were some linear progression of symptoms. People would sometimes ask me if my father was in stage 1 or stage 3. I'm not even sure how that form of assessment started, but I do know that it didn't last long. Those of us who were going through the experience of losing someone to Alzheimer's quickly realized such a notion was ridiculous. There are no clear lines delineating where a person is in the progression of dementia. But it's still valuable to think of the disease as having a beginning, a middle, and an end, even if the lines are vague. For one thing, it helps the caregiver figure out what needs to be dealt with and when.

❧

MANY YEARS AGO I had a friend who always used to say jokingly, "I hate change!" He would say it about small things as well as major events. After watching him through a few bouts of change, I started to doubt that he was joking. If he could have stopped time in its tracks, I believe he would have. To some degree, we all have a bit of that. We're creatures of habit. We don't like it when the landscape around us changes. When Alzheimer's takes over, it alters almost everything, with no warning and no predictability. If your tendency is to be controlling, you are in for a bumpy ride.

In the early stages, in those frantic moments after your worst fears have been confirmed, there are times when the person who has been diagnosed seems perfectly fine. They engage in coherent conversations, they cook dinner, they remember appointments. Then, with no warning, as if a thread has been snipped, they are different—confused, upset by their own confusion, incapable of remembering the simplest thing or of thinking logically. It's a bit of a roller-coaster ride, and there is simply no way to predict when they will be fine and when they will seem lost. The challenge is to adapt to the unpredictability early on; fighting it will only bring torment to everyone. I used to tell myself when I went to see my father that I didn't know what I was going to find, or how he was going to be, but I was willing to be open to whatever happened. I gained great reverence for those three words: I don't know.

Think about your own fears and panic around discovering that your loved one has dementia, and then multiply that by a hundred when you think about how they must feel. They've just been given a death sentence, but it's death by a thousand cuts. They will lose their memory, their identity—sometimes incrementally, sometimes in huge chunks. The future suddenly looks like a minefield. And no one can offer them hope for a cure because at the moment there isn't one. If you keep in mind that your loved one has to be racked with fear even if they aren't showing it, you will have opened the door to compassion regardless of what your relationship with them has been like.

♰

THE TONE THAT IS SET in the early stages will in all likelihood carry through for the rest of your journey, however long that is. It's a time when you need to be clear about where you're coming from, what emotions are at play, and how you are going to relate to your loved one now that you know they are traveling down a narrowing path, a path where you can't follow.

I've noticed that almost from the moment of diagnosis, there is a tendency to start talking to a dementia patient differently, in a slower cadence, emphasizing certain words much the same as we do when we speak to very young children. I caught myself doing that with my father the first time I flew back to Los Angeles from New York after his diagnosis was made public. It's something to be wary of because it can easily go too far—you can end up interacting with your loved one as if they no longer deserve to be treated with dignity. That can then veer into treating them as if they are invisible. Early in the disease you can still talk to them normally; you just may have to repeat yourself a few times.

It's important to address some very practical safety measures, which will then make you acutely aware of the necessary role reversal. You have to start acting like a parent to your parent, a strange and unfamiliar dance. Like taking away the car keys or insisting that your loved one cannot be left alone, some things are simply not negotiable.

If there are any weapons in the house, get rid of them, along with the ammunition. It's an individual choice whether or not to tell your loved one what you're doing, but there can be no bargaining on this. Kitchen items like knives should either be put out of reach or secured in a locked drawer. If your parent is still cooking, they should probably not be left unattended. The list of things that can go wrong and be dangerous is a lengthy one. We don't usually think about the locks on the inside doors of a home, particularly bathrooms. These should be removed, so loved ones cannot lock themselves in a bathroom, or any other room, and either refuse to come out or forget how to unlock the door. If there are tools, particularly power tools in the garage or basement, either get rid of them or lock them up. I heard about one man with Alzheimer's who took a chainsaw to the bedroom wall—he wanted a bigger room.

Making the home safe is sort of like childproofing on steroids. The things that a small child can get into are generally on the floor or several feet above. With a dementia patient, you have to think about what they can reach in a high cabinet. Don't fool yourself into thinking that they'll never pull up a chair and climb up to that shelf. Dementia doesn't wipe out the memories that have been encoded for a very long time, so it's reasonable to assume that they know perfectly well how to get to things that are out of reach.

❧

ONCE, EARLY IN MY father's illness, when I was still living in New York, I flew back to Los Angeles to visit him. We were sitting in the den in my parents' house, just me and my father, waiting for his doctor to come, which he did every two or three weeks. I remember we were talking about ice-skating—something I'd started to do every morning in Central Park—and my father was recounting how he used to ice-skate for hours on the frozen river when he was a kid. It was early afternoon, and he was alert and following the conversation.

When the doctor arrived, I noticed that he greeted my father in a loud, deliberate tone, slowing down his words as if he were speaking to someone who didn't understand English. I had never met this doctor before, and already I didn't like him. He then proceeded to talk about my father in the third person, as if he wasn't in the room.

Turning his attention to me, he said, "Since you don't live here and only visit occasionally, have you noticed any difference—any slippage in him—since the last time you were here?"

I think my jaw dropped. I was stunned at this man's callousness and I couldn't even find my voice at first. I was suddenly aware that my father was staring at me. I looked over at him and his eyes were laser-focused, boring into me with something very deliberate in them. I felt I knew what he was thinking: Let's see how she handles this. An ancient theme from childhood tugged at me—I wanted him to be proud of me. I also wanted to put this doctor in his place.

"My father is sitting right here. You're talking about him in third person. That hardly seems right," I told him.

Undeterred, the doctor continued. "He doesn't understand what we're talking about," he said, waving his hand dismissively. "Cognitively, he can't understand. He can still feel emotions, but his brain is not working the same. Now, you didn't answer my question."

"And I'm not going to answer your question when it's framed the way you framed it," I told him.

I honestly can't recall what was said next because I decided I was never again going to have a conversation with this doctor. The look in my father's eyes had turned amused; I believed then and believe now that he and I were communicating just fine. Our history leaned in on us—all the times I had hurt him, particularly when he was president, when I spoke out publicly against his policies. But now, in this quiet room in my parents' house, with late afternoon light spilling in and the cawing of a crow mingling with the sound of a far-away siren, I was defending his right to be treated with dignity. Behind the twinkle in his eyes, I knew he was thinking, Good girl, you got this exactly right. I reported to my mother what had happened and I wasn't surprised that shortly after that my father had a new doctor.

☙

MANY YEARS LATER, a little while after I had started the Beyond Alzheimer's support group, an older couple came in one night and sat down. They were a few minutes late, so we had already started, but I briefly interrupted the group member who was talking so I could get the newcomers' names and introduce myself and my cofacilitator. I had an uncomfortable feeling that the man had dementia. It was nothing overt, just a look in his eyes. The group was strictly for caregivers; it was a place for them to speak freely and openly, without their loved ones hearing them. I hoped I was wrong about this couple, but when we got around to them, the woman began speaking about her husband in third person—very harshly, I might add. She was talking about how he didn't understand things anymore and couldn't do simple tasks. Before I could stop her, a man in the group cut her off and said, "We're all very uncomfortable with this. You're speaking about your husband as if he isn't here, but he's right next to you."

"He doesn't understand what I'm saying," she snapped.

At that point my cofacilitator took the man, who was very sweet and who I believe understood exactly what he was hearing, out of the room and waited with him in the hallway while we first explained to this woman that the group was not for patients. More importantly, we then tried to explain that it is not helpful and can in fact be unkind to do what she was doing—talking about him as if he wasn't present. I don't think any of it got through to her and we never saw her again.

I tell these two stories to show how extreme the attitude of "They don't understand anything" can get. I'm afraid this is all too common, and even if things aren't as glaring as the examples I've given, milder versions can still do damage. I wanted to say to that woman, "Your husband is still a human being!" I didn't, but I remember how my hands shook. The dismissive attitude, which she had in spades, is something to be conscious of because it can sneak up on even the kindest people. You see that distant look in your loved one's eyes, you know they're far away, and you feel you don't know them anymore. You assume it doesn't matter what you say in their presence. It does matter, though. From the early stages until the end, it matters.

Years ago, it was assumed that people in a coma couldn't hear anything, so it didn't matter what you said when you were standing in the room. It's not dissimilar to how some people regard Alzheimer's patients. Even the most conventional doctors will say now that we have no idea what a comatose person might be picking up on. So, whoever is near them needs to be careful about what they say. In the same way, none of us knows what a person with Alzheimer's is absorbing.

✑

IN THE FIRST YEAR of my father's illness I met a woman who told me that her grandmother had recently died from Alzheimer's. She was actually one of the first people who talked to me in some detail about the disease. She told me that she had never particularly liked her grandmother—the woman was very closed off, not loving or affectionate at all. If she asked her parents why, they would say something cryptic like, "She had a hard life." Which, of course, didn't explain much. From an early point in the disease, her grandmother started traveling back in time to when she was a young girl—in Germany, in the 1940s. She, along with her parents, were put into a crowded train and taken to Auschwitz. Her parents died there; she barely survived. And the rest of her life was haunted by memories that never dimmed.

It was heartbreaking, this woman told me, to listen to her grandmother, who was reliving the concentration camp. The horrors, the nightmare, the stench of death, and the grip of terror were absolutely real to her. There was nothing anyone could do except listen and learn and wait for Alzheimer's to move her down the road to another time period. She understood then why her grandmother wouldn't let anyone get close to her, why she was so closed off.

I've thought of that story often. I'm so grateful I heard it in the beginning stages of my father's illness because it was like a lantern I carried with me to cut through the shadows. It was my reminder to stay open and not be trapped by any past decisions or judgments.

Obviously, my father had nothing so dramatic in his past, but I did get to know, as the years unspooled and he moved back through time, the boy who decided he was going to have a sturdier, more dependable life than his father. The boy who dreamed beyond the small towns they moved to every time his father lost another job, and the hardscrabble life of wondering which bills could wait and which had to be paid, of worrying whether there would be enough food for the week ahead. My father grew up with uncertainty—that's how it is when you live with an alcoholic—but he refused to accept uncertainty as his fate. In a way, his sights were always set past his immediate circumstances; he was always aiming for higher ground. The feeling I had growing up—that he was looking past me to something bigger, more important, was right. I just didn't fully understand where it came from until he started leaving.

❧

FROM EARLY ON IN the disease caregivers tend to start limiting their own lives—eliminating fun, joy, respite. Countless people in my support group describe how constricted their lives have become and, when asked how this happened, say something like, "Well, my father (or mother, or spouse, or partner) can't go out and have fun . . . " The interesting thing is, that they generally never finish the sentence. If you put into words what the rest of that thought is, the absence of logic is glaring.

"So, then, you shouldn't have any fun or pleasure because they can't?" either my cofacilitator or I would say. Sometimes I would also point out that, yes, your loved one is ill and it's a serious, terminal illness, but you didn't give him or her dementia. So how does self-punishment make any sense? Usually when people hear it put into language, they get it, at least intellectually. But that doesn't necessarily mean their behavior, and how they treat themselves, will instantly change. The notion of sacrifice is something we hold onto subconsciously, and the subconscious is stubborn. The problem is that we confuse self-care with neglect for the person who is ill. We have a misguided notion that if we are out having a good time, we're shirking our responsibilities as caregivers, and somehow being disloyal and uncaring.

It's a good idea to clarify what neglect is. If you fail to provide adequate care for a loved one with dementia, if you leave them alone and don't take steps to minimize risk, you are being neglectful. But if your loved one has appropriate supervision, if hazardous things around the house like knives and tools are locked away, if you've taken the car keys and hopefully the car as well . . . how does it make sense to sacrifice joy and fun in your own life?

The analogy I'm fond of using is this: When you're on a plane, the preflight announcement instructs, "If the oxygen masks drop and you're traveling with a child or someone who needs assistance, put your own mask on first." We've all heard this over and over, but we do not analyze exactly why it's important. If you're fighting for breath, you are not going to be able to help another person. Similarly, if you are suffocating under the weight of self-sacrifice and restriction, you aren't going to be your best as a caregiver. You might follow every tip, every suggestion for how to deal with the situations that come up, but if your spirit is depleted and your health run down, that advice probably won't work well. The energy you bring to caregiving, just like everything else in your life, goes a long way in determining the results.

It always fascinated me when a new person came into the support group and started talking about why they were there. They gave detailed descriptions of their loved one's diagnosis and condition, often reading from their notes about medications and physicians' comments. We would let them finish and then say, "So how are *you* doing?" Almost every time, the attendee was shocked. No one had asked them before. People would always ask how their loved one was, but never inquire about them. It often took an adjustment period for them to accept that they mattered too, that they were part of the equation, and their life deserved to be nurtured and cared for as well.

❧

IN THE EARLY STAGES of dementia it's important for the family to address topics that they might not be able to discuss later, when their loved one no longer has periods of lucidity. Now is the time to have conversations about financial matters, wills, end-of-life wishes.

It's never easy to talk about death. But it will come for all of us, and it's important to know what your loved one's wishes are. Maybe they have already documented their preferences years earlier; if so, you need to confirm that whatever they stated then is still what they want. If they chose a DNR (Do Not Resuscitate) order, you should know where it is and make sure it's accessible. If an unexpected event happens—a fall, a heart attack, a stroke—and paramedics come, they will not take your word that a DNR exists. If they don't have a copy in hand, they will use every method available to save the person's life. One of the cofacilitators in my support group used to suggest that the DNR be taped to the refrigerator. That might be too disturbing for some people, but you can understand the point.

Who is going to have medical power of attorney? This may be tricky. Sometimes a spouse is not the best person to take on this responsibility, even though it may seem like the logical choice. If, for example, your mother doesn't want to be resuscitated, wants to be allowed to die under circumstances made clear in the DNR, your father might not be fully behind that idea, and therefore isn't the best person to carry out her wishes. It's an important decision, and one that needs to be made when the person who has dementia has the clarity to make it. The decision can cause tension between siblings— why does he or she get that role and I don't? It's a good idea for everyone to acknowledge that decisions about death and dying are personal, intimate matters, and every individual has the right to make the choice that feels right to them. Jealousies and ruffled feelings have no place there.

At the moment, eight states have a Death with Dignity law that allows euthanasia to be utilized when a person is terminally ill and does not want to suffer anymore.[1] There is an exception to who can request this, though: people with dementia. Anyone who wishes it to be invoked must establish and document the choice before a diagnosis of dementia. However, there are now three advance directives for Alzheimer's in the United States that lay out some of the specific concerns of those with the disease, like feeding and palliative care in the latter stages.[2] So, some progress is being made to give dementia patients a say in how many or how few life-prolonging measures they want.

Recently, there have been news reports about people in care facilities who requested the withdrawal of food, water, and some palliative care when they reach the end stages of dementia and were denied that by the facility. A story in the *Washington Post* detailed one woman's struggle with the facility she called home.[3] The facility cited its policies of continuing to give food and especially water until the moment of death, and one administrator was quoted as saying that he felt he knew best if someone really wants to be given sustenance, no matter what that person designated in a written directive. This has happened in other facilities as well. Some family members have, in the face of this kind of denial, actually removed their loved ones from the facilities and taken them home to honor the wishes that were expressed.

If your loved one is in a facility, find out ahead of time what its rules and procedures are and plan accordingly.

End-of-life conversations are difficult to have, but they're necessary. The mother of a woman I know had refused to do anything along these lines, and when her health declined to the point where life-and-death decisions had to be made, her daughter was left with the daunting task of trying to intuit what her mother would want. Lack of preparation made a painful situation even more painful.

Some of our trepidation about bringing up the subject of death and end-of-life wishes has to do with feelings we harbor within ourselves. It actually may not be daunting at all for someone who has just received a terminal diagnosis of dementia to talk about death. Family members or spouses, on the other hand, may be reluctant to go there. What's at play are their own fears. Once again, dementia hands caregivers an opportunity to unearth feelings they have avoided for years.

Fear of death has taken up a lot of space in my life. It started when I was a child: I clearly remember lying in bed at age six or seven and talking to God about being scared to die. I was fixated on this because I was painfully aware of how annoyed my mother seemed to be by my presence, so I decided God must have made a mistake in sending me into the world. Surely, I thought, He would realize His mistake and then He'd have to take me back. I tried to console myself with the stories my father told me about heaven and how beautiful it was, but fear sat cold and immovable in me. As I got older, I pushed that fear down so I wouldn't have to think about it.

I have met two people who had no fear of death. Both had experienced accidents in which they "died" and then came back. One of them was a caregiver who came to my support group; the calmness and acceptance she showed when the subject of death came up was infectious. I literally watched people's facial expressions change and get smoother, more relaxed. The other woman, whom I had met many years before, told me something that has stayed with me. She said that, initially, when she "came back," she didn't want to be here. What she'd seen was so beautiful, this world held little interest for her. A friend finally confronted her and said, "You were brought back here to be present in this world, not to just bide your time until you die . . . again. You came back so that you could show up. So, start showing up." Those words changed her life. And when I heard this, I thought maybe some of our fear about death is actually a fear about life. The fear that we didn't do enough, love enough, give enough back, that the mistakes we've made can never be forgiven. I think, if we are going to look clearly at our own fear of death, we also have to look clearly at how we view the life we have lived.

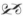

A COMPLICATING FACTOR IN the early stages of Alzheimer's is that the people who are ill still have enough cognition to want things that have always been constants in their life. They assume they can do what they've done before. Like travel. This is going to be tricky.

If there are relatives who live far away, who your loved one wants to visit, or there is someplace they have always wanted to go, you need to do that before the disease worsens. Travel is extremely risky for people with dementia, so it's a judgment call whether they are still able to handle it at this stage. Later on, I can assure you, they will not be able to. The crowds at airports, the unpredictability of air travel, and all the things that can go wrong are disorienting and can easily lead to panic. If you do manage to get them to the destination without incident, being in an unfamiliar environment, perhaps in a different time zone, is going to be a problem. With Alzheimer's, the world gets smaller—at least the world one is comfortable inhabiting. So, a change of environment becomes frightening. It may be possible for individuals to travel and keep things smooth in the very early stages of the disease, but it's something to be cautious about.

My father never went on a plane again after his diagnosis, but he and my mother would still go up to the ranch he loved in Refugio Canyon, north of Santa Barbara. It's about a two-hour drive, and once you get into the canyon, the road up to the ranch is a steep hill of switchbacks. It's narrow—barely two lanes—a scary road for anyone. I can't imagine what it's like for someone with Alzheimer's. But for a while, the visits went fine. Then came a day when they set out on the Coast Highway, heading north, and my father began to panic. Two Secret Service agents were in the front of the car and my parents were in the back. According to my mother's account, my father was disoriented, couldn't figure out where they were or where they were going, and nothing anyone said could calm him down. She called me from the ranch later and told me that his upset continued even when they got there. It broke my heart. This man who loved vast open spaces, who lived for riding his horse to the top of hills and looking down at the Pacific Ocean and the green swaths of land between, was now desperate to go back to the section of the house he was most familiar with. All that open space frightened him, as if he had never seen it before, as if he had never loved it and needed it to feed his soul. He never went to the ranch again.

These were years when people were not speaking openly about

Alzheimer's; I mentally marked this as a lesson learned, and assumed my father was not the only person with the disease whose world was growing steadily smaller. Now, of course, I know that's true. Pay attention to, and watch out for this development, because it will happen. It's one of the few predictable symptoms of Alzheimer's.

In later years, when my father had drifted far away, I would sometimes look at his eyes and hope that wherever he had traveled to inside himself was a place that resembled what he had always loved—green and vast, with wind brushing across the hillsides and his horse strong beneath him, hooves sharp and sure on the ground, ready to take him wherever he wanted to go. There was something peaceful about his countenance in those late stages, as if he had tapped into something the rest of us couldn't see.

"It is those we live with and love and should know who elude us."   —NORMAN MACLEAN, *A River Runs Through It*

CHAPTER 5

Time Warp

Worlds evolve inside houses. Even after we have moved out of our family home and have established our own independent lives, the life we lived inside those walls remains with us, living inside us, pulling at us even when we aren't aware of it.

A man who grew up under the shadow of his older brother always felt dwarfed and insignificant. His father had heaped praise on his brother but withheld affection from him. As an adult, he struggles to find self-confidence. Then he learns that his father has Alzheimer's. He doesn't know now how to relate to his parent in the face of a diminishing disease that will steal everything in the end. The father was a towering figure who had made his son feel small; now that son watches helplessly as his father seems to shrink. Where does he fit now as a son? What's his place in this new reality? Will he be able to take his place alongside his brother, or will he still be left behind—the boy who always felt he was an afterthought?

A woman's father drank his way through her childhood, turning their family home into a scene of rage and nightmare. Decades later, he is diagnosed with dementia. As an adult, the daughter has avoided him, holding fast to resentment over the memories that still burn in her. Is she supposed to forgive him now? Tend to him? She doesn't know. She's ten years old again, crouched in her bedroom closet, waiting for the yelling to stop.

A woman whose mother was always her best friend, steering her through rough times and celebrating her joys and successes, now sees that her mother can't remember what happened yesterday. Part of her believed her mother would always be there. The loneliness feels vast and terrifying. How is she to navigate her way through life without her?

All these situations are different, but they are tethered by the commonality of seeing a parent slipping into the distance and getting caught in a time warp. Suddenly, grown sons and daughters are propelled back into childhood, into the relationship that defined their earliest years. They're facing adult challenges—the illness of a parent and in this case the unpredictability of dementia—yet emotionally a twelve-year-old self is saying, "What about me?"

This shocks a lot of people who thought they had worked through their parental issues, either in therapy or with diligent self-work. But Alzheimer's has a way of rooting out what has lain dormant for years. You thought you'd forgiven your parent for exiling you when you came out to them and told them you were gay? Guess what—some old resentment lingers there. And now you face the prospect of having to care for that parent in ways they didn't for you.

The daughter whose mother was there when she delivered her

baby, who helped her through the daunting challenges of new motherhood, who has been a hands-on grandmother, is certain that she has outgrown her dependence. She appreciates all her mother does and their closeness, but she feels grounded in adulthood. She no longer identifies with the needy girl she once was—until her mother can't remember how to load the washing machine. Then that grown daughter is young again, needing to cry in her mother's arms, except it's her mother who now needs comforting. The role reversal is almost too much to bear.

It's difficult to be flung backward through time; instinct wants us to move forward, believing that childhood and adolescence are merely images in the rearview mirror. But the world of dementia is full of mirrors. So . . . what to do? The options are fairly basic. You can see it as a punishment, or as an opportunity. The child or the adolescent who has broken out of his or her hiding place and is now intruding on your psyche is doing it because that incarnation still has something to tell you. They'll settle down only if you listen.

We owe it to ourselves to explore the history that lingers in us—not out of self-pity, not to validate the ways in which we were victims, but to see more clearly how pieces of our past are cluttering up the present. Our twelve-year-old self won't be able to adequately care for a parent with Alzheimer's. No matter how diligently we follow advice and practical methods of care, if our emotional identity is rooted in childhood paradigms, it's not going to work. One of the many lessons that Alzheimer's teaches us is that it's time to grow up.

❧

I'VE HEARD A NUMBER of people say, usually about a parent with whom they had a difficult relationship, "I have some things I want to tell them before they're too far gone to understand," or some version of that. Usually when people bring this up they elaborate on exactly what it is they want to confront their parent with. But they really don't need to elaborate—their tone says everything. I understand the desire to declare the ways in which a parent has hurt you; it feels as if you're standing up for yourself, setting the record straight. And I get that there is a long-buried wish that maybe that parent will apologize, make amends. I've been there, too. But the truth is, if they haven't apologized by this point, they probably aren't going to now. You might think that you have never told them about your grievances, and it's important that they know. But most of us have made clear to our parents in one way or another exactly what we resent them for. At a certain point in our lives, the details of what happened in the past don't matter. What matters is that we're still invested in the grievances.

You will never learn the lessons that Alzheimer's can teach if you're still locked inside your own history. I've heard terrible stories about how a son or daughter was treated by a parent—tales of physical and emotional violence, deliberate cruelty, banishment because of sexual orientation, even threats made with weapons. Then that parent is diagnosed with dementia. There is an opportunity here to walk away from the past and bolt the doors behind you. You won't forget what happened but you don't have to reside there. As dementia claims your parent, you might learn a lot about how they came to be that person, and that's the doorway to forgiveness.

✑

WHEN I GOT THE news of my father's diagnosis, one of my earliest thoughts was that I had to get this right. I'd gotten so many things wrong in my life, especially with my family, I *had* to get this one right.

It's not the worst thought, but I knew I was weighed down by my past—especially when it came to my parents. I felt that much of what had gone wrong in my family was probably my fault, even though, truthfully, there was plenty of blame to go around. I was in my forties, but part of me was still the sulking, self-conscious teenager sent off to boarding school with not a lot of friends. The girl who seemed to fumble her way through life. I knew I couldn't simply tell that girl to shut up and go away; I had to deal with her. I had to figure out why she felt like that, but from the perspective of an adult who had learned some things along the way and who was, in fact, fully capable of being a grown-up.

We all make decisions about ourselves, starting way back in childhood. We see ourselves a certain way in the mirror, and often that reflection doesn't change as we grow up. It takes resolve to look back, understand the decisions we made, and work on changing them. In 1994, when this strange disease entered my family's life, I knew that was exactly the work I needed to do.

I thought about how ours was a different kind of home than the ones I walked into when I had playdates—homes where the kids were at the center of everything and the rest of life sort of revolved around them. Our home had a different homeostasis to it. I knew my parents loved me and my brother, but we hovered just outside the circle of their bright life. It was a circle we could never really penetrate, and in the clear-eyed intuition of children, we knew it. I thought about the nearsighted adolescent who kept to herself because she didn't think she was pretty enough or fun enough to be included in any of the cliques that always form in schools, who ran track and kept her nose buried in books. I was fine by myself. I thought about the nineteen-year-old, away at college, who sat in a dark bathroom in the dead of night, the glow of a streetlight filling up a corner of the window. I held a razor blade against the soft veins of my wrist and thought how easy it would be if I just pressed harder. I was ravaged by the amphetamines I'd become addicted to in an attempt to be thin and accepted. But no matter how thin I got, or how hard I tried, I felt invisible. It was an echo of my father's voice that saved me from taking my life that winter night. He used to tell me that God put everyone here for a reason, that He never made mistakes and that He loved all His children. I put the razor blade down because I didn't want God to be disappointed in me.

In 1994 I realized that I had bundled up the perceptions that I was not good enough, not worth much, that I was the one who always got in trouble, got things wrong, didn't fit in, and I had carried that bundle with me for decades. I was never going to "get it right" in dealing with my father's Alzheimer's if I was still lugging around my bundle of self-doubt and defeat. Unfortunately, it isn't just something you can drop and walk away from; this metaphorical knapsack had attached itself to my brain cells. I knew I literally had to rewire my brain.

I started trying to catch myself every time a negative, self-punishing thought intruded, like "I'm going to mess this up," or "I'm never going to be successful in this," or "I'm such an idiot." I had a friend at that time who used to say, "The subconscious has no sense of humor, so be careful what messages you give it." I realized that even if I was half joking when I called myself an idiot, my subconscious was putting that in its hard drive, and not as a joke. I decided on this method: whenever the old paradigm pushed its way in, I said to it, "Thanks for sharing. But I don't need you right now. I'm going in a different direction."

The decisions we've made about ourselves go all the way back to childhood; we've cemented them into the foundation of who we think we are. Changing them requires commitment and patience. It also requires forgiving ourselves when we slide back into the person we used to be, a person who will always be familiar to us but isn't necessarily the person we are capable of being.

In Alcoholics Anonymous they say, "It's easier to act your way into a new way of thinking than it is to think your way into a new way of acting." It's a valuable tip—pretend to be strong, capable, calm, and your emotions will catch up. If you don't think you're together enough or strong enough to handle the unpredictable turns of a loved one with Alzheimer's, just act as though you are. Do it enough, and you'll get there.

When I felt myself slipping, I made myself think of people whose confidence I admired, who were centered and together no matter what life threw at them (or at least that's how they appeared to me). I thought of their posture, the cadence of their voice, their body language when they spoke, and I tried to work on adapting those qualities. As an example, when I get scared and insecure, my shoulders rise up toward my ears and my spine curves. If I felt that happening, I thought of Beyoncé—it's basically impossible to imagine her slumping.

When I flew back to Los Angeles from New York to visit my father, I could more easily master the paradigm shift I was aiming for when I was alone with him. Sitting with him as evening moved into the sky, or taking a walk with him in the afternoon, I could master a sense of confidence that would ground me and make me more alert to what was going on with him. I believed that whatever Alzheimer's had in store, I could trust my instincts and deal with it in a way that would, I hoped, be soothing to my father and illuminating for me. And if I felt my confidence flagging, I'd think of the AA approach and visualize someone who would handle the situation calmly and insightfully. I'd straighten my spine, drop my shoulders from up around my ears, believing that eventually my emotional muscles would get used to it and say, "Hey, this feels pretty good."

The challenge came when I was with my mother. So much of my insecurity was tied to my relationship with her. Silencing my self-judgments was hard beneath her leveling stare. I knew I had the tools, but I didn't always rise to the task of using them. My mother knew right where my buttons were, and she was very adept at pushing them. It had, after all, been a lifetime dance between us. I had to remind myself to look at her as a woman whose life was completely wrapped up in her husband, who was now losing him in cruel and unpredictable ways. My role, as I saw it, was to try and mother her during such a painful chapter of her life, which was difficult since she had never shown much interest in mothering me.

I can think of many occasions when I fell short of my goal, but there were also many times when I got it right. One day my mother was particularly agitated and told me that my father was going to have a small basal cell growth removed from his face. She said she was afraid he wouldn't understand what was going on and would panic. She had tried to tell him, but he got confused and upset. With uncommon patience I reminded her that this was a precancerous growth and it would take many, many years to worsen into something serious. As she nodded, I tentatively pointed out that he was at that time eighty-six, with a terminal illness, and didn't have that many years left, so why put him through an unnecessary procedure that would undoubtedly frighten and confuse him? My mother could easily have lashed out at me, but miraculously she didn't. She ultimately agreed that it wasn't necessary, and even thanked me for my advice, which was a first. I was pretending to be calm and patient when inside I was terrified that my mother would explode in anger. I walked away from that moment thinking maybe I could actually accomplish this growing-up thing.

ABOUT TWO YEARS AFTER my father's Alzheimer's was made public, I moved back to Los Angeles from New York. I couldn't afford to keep flying back and forth across the country, and I wanted to spend time with my father, so I left the city that had been my home for a little over four years. I flew straight into my own turbulent history. My mother and I had fallen into another pit of tension, which meant it wasn't very comfortable for me to visit my father at my parents' home. But he was still going to his office in Century City during the week. I would go there to visit him. My brother Michael did as well. It was a chance to have some private time with our father, to listen to him and figure out the best ways to communicate as his thoughts and language became increasingly fragmented.

At a certain point, something odd started to happen. I would arrive at the building, where I had to check in downstairs with security, and when the guard called up to the office, he was told that my father either wasn't there or that he was too busy to see me. Not being there was a ridiculous claim—the Secret Service car was parked outside. And I knew perfectly well that even if he had a visitor—and the office staff did schedule some appointments—it would not be a long visit. By then, they were keeping these very short. Michael encountered the same thing. We both knew immediately what was going on. My mother had told them not to let us up. It was a control game, and a tactic that we were all too familiar with. When I was nineteen and moved out of my parents' house, she had prevented Ron, who at thirteen was still at home, from finding out where I was. Michael had frequently been excluded, kept at a distance, as had Maureen. Separation was a form of currency in my family.

Now we discussed what to do, and decided to tell Ron about it, since my mother tended to relinquish her desire for control when he was involved. What happened next was unprecedented. Ron flew down from Seattle and the three of us went to the house to speak with our mother (Michael's stepmother) while our father was at the office. We had never been a united front before, and I was acutely aware of how disorienting it was for my mother. As we began voicing our complaint, I realized that we probably didn't need to say anything. The very fact that we were sitting in front of her—three siblings with the same purpose—was all we needed to make our point. She attempted to make excuses or denials, but she was on such unfamiliar ground that she really didn't know what to say. I let myself bask in the fact that Ron, Michael, and I were behaving like a family, something we had never done before. If it never happened again, at least I would know that we had bonded on this one morning as sunlight streamed through the window and fell on the chair that was still our father's favorite place to sit.

Then I realized something else. Losing my father to Alzheimer's had so fractured my mother's world that it was a survival instinct to reach for what was most familiar, which in this case was separation and power play. That was the rope she grabbed onto to keep from drowning. I gained a great deal of compassion for my mother that morning as I let myself consider what was at work on the deeper levels of her emotions. Predictably, we were never turned away from our father's office again. But I am convinced that if I had gone into that visit blinded by the past, I wouldn't have seen the things I saw; I wouldn't have changed my perspective and looked beneath my mother's actions to the grief that she didn't know what to do with.

WE DON'T CHANGE IN a linear pattern. There are leaps ahead, there are stumbles, and there are times we fall backward. That's particularly true when it comes to family dynamics.

There is a line in the book *A Course in Miracles*: "Do you want to be right or do you want to be at peace?"[4] Over time it became clear to me that if I asked myself that question when it came to my mother, sometimes the truth was, "I want to be right. Forget about peace right now, I'm going to dig my heels in here." After I backslid, I would realize that then I had chosen to be fourteen, or eighteen, or whatever age I was planted in.

That was definitely an Aha! moment for me, and years later I was able to pass it along to people in my support group who sometimes talked about how they fell back into old behavior patterns with a parent or sibling. They felt guilty about it, as if they had lost a race that they had spent a lot of time training for. In offering the quote from *A Course in Miracles*, I'd suggest to them that whether you want to be at peace or be right is an important question to ask, but there is no wrong answer. If what you really want is to be right at that moment, then own that decision and be clear about it. Next time around you might choose differently. Just know what ground you're standing on.

I heard a story long ago about Carl Jung and one of his patients who said to him, regarding whatever issues he or she was wrestling with, "I'm so tired of this." Jung replied, "Good. Now we can get to work."

The best thing that can happen to us is that we get tired of our childish or adolescent ways. There were times during my father's Alzheimer's when I was not acting like a woman in her forties—mostly when I was around my mother. The energy I was expending exhausted me. Eventually, that insecure, angry eighteen-year-old didn't feel like a good fit anymore. Alzheimer's was my teacher. It's a harsh teacher, and learning comes at great emotional cost, but it can help you stretch into the person you were always meant to be.

Dealing with Alzheimer's, or any kind of dementia, is like nothing else. You can't compare it to having a loved one with cancer, or even Lou Gehrig's disease (ALS), as devastating as those are. Those afflicted with such diseases can still think linear thoughts; they can still remember, and they can still interact. Dementia is a landscape of unmarked trails. No one knows what's going to happen next; the only certainty is that it's going to get worse. To approach dementia still clinging to adolescent ways is not going to serve you well. Navigating your way through the maze of dementia requires the steadiness of a grown-up. Like many unexpected challenges in life, Alzheimer's is a wake-up call to let go of childish ways and step into the world of adulthood.

❧

ANOTHER THING AT PLAY here sends us spiraling back to who we used to be—denial. Denial of the disease and its impact, as well as its inevitable end stages. If we stay locked in the dynamic of a parent pushing our buttons and get upset in all the ways we used to, then it's almost as if time has gone backward. We're young again, we're caught in the same familiar theatrics, we're miles away from the present moment with a devastating illness bearing down on us. Denial is a tantalizing escape method, one that we all have an aptitude for.

No one is wrong, or to blame, for slipping into the mind-set of a younger self. It just means you're human. But your journey with Alzheimer's is going to be defined by how willing you are to change and look at things from another angle.

The thirteenth-century Persian poet Rumi said, "As you live deeper in the heart, the mirror gets clearer and cleaner." So much of the experience of dealing with dementia is about what's going on in the heart, or at least it should be. If you stay with that, things do ultimately get clearer. Not at first, and usually not for a while, but in time there is a parting of the shadows, and a light that illuminates everything—your relationship with the person who is leaving, your history with them, the dreams that were realized and the hopes that got trampled. It's humbling, this disease. It makes us acutely aware of how complicated we are, how strong we can be, and how vulnerable we need to be.

When you are dealing with the first stages of the disease, it's helpful to find some kind of support system, whether it's a group, or a few trusted friends, even a pastor or counselor—someone with whom you can speak honestly and openly. Because everything is so new, and the unpredictability of dementia can be overwhelming, having a safety net from the start is important, having someone who can point out your denial and show you a way past it. If you can't find someone in your life to talk to, the Alzheimer's Association has a twenty-four-hour hotline.[5] It is going to be a lonely journey, but there are ways to make it less lonely.

Someone said to me, shortly after his parent was diagnosed, that he was looking for a guiding star. The thing about stars is they can only be seen in the dark.

"The only wisdom we can hope to acquire is the wisdom of humility."
                                          —T. S. Eliot, "Four Quartets"

MESSY EMOTIONS
AND LEARNING TO LIE

CHAPTER 6

Caregiver Stress

"Fight or flight" refers to the adrenalized state that fear triggers in us. We were given the fear response as a means of survival. Many stories are told of people lifting cars off trapped children, running on broken legs, fighting off attackers with strength they did not possess in their daily lives. In *The Gift of Fear*, security expert Gavin de Becker explored the instinct that arises when we sense danger—often before our brains have processed what's going on.[1] He emphasized the importance of listening to that instinct, trusting it, because it can literally save our lives.

But the fight-or-flight response is meant to play out in a relatively short amount of time. Physiologically, the hormones that are released, including adrenaline, are supposed to settle again to normal levels after thirty or forty minutes. Hanging onto our fear, recycling it through our brains until it becomes like background music, turns into chronic stress.

Stress is often at the root of many health problems caregivers face. In fact, the term "caregiver stress" evolved because doctors kept encountering the toll that caregiving takes on human health—heart issues, recurrent viruses, sleep disorders, breathing problems. Even frequent accidents can be a symptom of stress. It occurs when fear is not reasonable, is not there for your survival but is instead damaging you. And it happens a lot with Alzheimer's.

A common fear is that there is a genetic predisposition to the disease. Some people constantly worry about whether they are going to get dementia because a parent has it; others have simply decided that this is their fate. Both of these mind-sets translate to stress.

Facts are important. One fact is that there is only one disease which you will absolutely get if you have the gene for it, and that's Huntington's Chorea.[2] While the offspring of someone with Huntington's Chorea have a 50 percent chance of inheriting the gene, if they have inherited it, it is 100 percent certain that they will get the disease. It doesn't matter if they live the healthiest life imaginable: if they possess the gene for Huntington's Chorea, that will be their fate unless they die of something else first. Every other disease is a matter of percentages, and that is not an exact science because lifestyle choices are a big factor.

A version of early-onset Alzheimer's typically shows up as a constant from one generation to the next. In this form of Alzheimer's, at least one person in each generation has been diagnosed with the disease before age sixty-five. If that's the case in your family as you look back through generations, there is a reason to be concerned. But even that situation doesn't come with any definitive predictions, and living in a constant state of stress caused by fear is a risky way to live.

Since I am not a scientist, I am not going to get into scientific gene studies. What I am going to discuss is how to handle the information that's available to us. Getting information online is a double-edged sword—you can end up more knowledgeable, but you can also end up terrified.

The conventional wisdom about everyone's risk for Alzheimer's is that, by the age of eighty, you have a 50/50 chance of getting the disease. I've said that to people and watched them get pale and frightened. All they've heard is the 50 percent chance that they might get Alzheimer's, not the 50 percent chance that they won't. Our imaginations can career in wild directions; we can decide that horrible fates await us. It's up to us to tame those thoughts and realize there is no benefit to panicking. In fact, there is a big downside to it. The author Deepak Chopra is famous for saying that the cells in our bodies listen to the cells in our brains. Obsessing over the fear of a disease that you *might* get creates an environment of stress in your body that can manifest in some kind of health problem. Maybe you won't get the exact disease you've been worrying about, but if stress is corroding your body's immune system, you've made yourself vulnerable to a variety of disorders.

Dr. Joe Dispenza has written numerous books on the connection between the brain and the body and has given many lectures that can be found online. He has backed up his philosophy with extensive scientific research, and I urge you to look him up and learn from him.[3] Here is a story he told in *You Are the Placebo* that dramatically emphasizes the power our thoughts and memories have over us:

In 1984, Gretchen van Boemel, MD, was practicing at the Doheny Eye Institute in Los Angeles when she began to see a large number of Cambodian women, all living in a Long Beach community known as Little Phnom Penh, who were having severe eye problems, including blindness. Strangely, when van Boemel examined their eyes, she found nothing wrong; their eyes were healthy. She did brain scans, and still could not explain why women whose visual acuity was 20/20 or better presented as nearly blind.

She teamed up with Patricia Rozée, PhD, at California State University in Long Beach to do research on the women. What they found was that the women, all between the ages of forty and sixty, had survived the brutality of the Khmer Rouge when the dictator Pol Pot was in power. Many of them had lost all their family members; many had been forced to watch as their loved ones were slaughtered. One woman who watched as her husband and four children were murdered in front of her lost her eyesight immediately. Another woman witnessed a Khmer Rouge soldier beating her brother and his children to death, killing her three-month-old nephew by repeatedly throwing him against a tree. She began losing her eyesight right afterward. The women were starved, beaten, sexually molested, humiliated, and tortured. They admitted to nightmares and flashbacks—a loop of the traumatizing events constantly playing in their minds. Van Boemel and Rozée documented numerous cases of psychosomatic blindness in the Cambodian women of this Long Beach community. Results of the study were presented at the 1986 American Psychological Association annual meeting in Washington, D.C.[4] The women were not blind because of any physical ailment or disease. The emotional effect of witnessing such horror and brutality made them not want to see anymore. And the replaying of those events in their minds meant their vision couldn't improve.

This is obviously an extreme example of how stress can affect us physically, but it demonstrates how our bodies listen to our minds, how ailments and illnesses can be caused by traumatic experiences. Stress is, at its root, fear. And constantly being in fear scrapes away at us.

I am hardly a stranger to fear. Anyone who knows me will attest to that. If I get the sniffles, I think I might have nose cancer. But I have never been frightened that I would get Alzheimer's, and that's because I made a very firm decision early on. I resolved to never let my fear attach itself to the notion of getting the disease. So far, it has worked. I believe we all have much more control over our fears than we give ourselves credit for.

When I moved back to California from New York, I rented a small, funky apartment on the beach in Malibu, thinking that maybe being near the ocean would make me feel closer emotionally to my father. He was several years into Alzheimer's at that point and he wasn't allowed to swim anymore—a decision I very much wanted to argue against, but I kept my mouth shut. I thought it was highly unlikely that he would forget how to swim and sink under the water, but I would have had to argue with my mother and my father's doctor, and I would have lost.

In a strange way, I felt like I was swimming for him. At my beach home I would plunge into the surf, swim past the breaking waves, and imagine his voice shouting, "Swim!" as a huge wave crested behind me, the way he did in long-ago summers, when I learned a lot about reining in my worst thoughts. I was scared of the big waves, but I wanted to be with my father. I wanted him to be proud of my athleticism, so I pushed past my fear and swam as hard as I could. I'd end up riding a wave to shore just behind him, his smile waiting for me as I scrambled to my feet, and in that moment, with him beaming at me, my fear was just a tiny shape drifting somewhere behind me in a vast ocean.

My new home on the beach was small and creaky and old, but I loved being on the water. When I walked along the shore, I would pass a wealthier stretch of beach, dotted with huge mansions, and I frequently ran into a man I knew who was in the film industry. He would always stop and ask my how my father was, and then talk to me about his mother, who also had Alzheimer's.

"I'm not even sure why I visit her," he would say. "She really isn't here anymore. She doesn't know I'm visiting her."

I would tell him about the belief that was shepherding me through every visit, every moment with my father—the belief that his soul didn't have Alzheimer's. Every single time, this man would cut off the conversation at that exact point, say goodbye, and walk off along the shore. I finally had to accept that he was never going to be open to what I had to say. So, I began to just listen to him, and not offer any counterpoint to what he was telling me. The other thread that ran through his conversation was an absolute certainty that he was going to get Alzheimer's because his mother had it. I desperately wanted to try to talk him out of this conviction, but I figured that wouldn't work out any better than my previous attempt to influence him. I kept my mouth shut and listened. Years later, I learned that he had been diagnosed with Alzheimer's.

I was horrified one evening when someone in my support group said she had learned through an online company that she had the APOE gene and was at risk for Alzheimer's. I had no idea at the time that this company was offering genetic as well as ancestry profiles, and I was stunned. We are all vulnerable to suggestion, and for a company to send frightening information with no counseling, no explanation of the entire picture, is in my opinion shockingly irresponsible. If you want to find out more about your great-great-grandparents, go for it. But you might want to think twice about sending off your saliva to a company that may tell you something disturbing.

I don't know anyone who is strong enough to set aside information like this and live their life as if they have never heard it. Whether you worry about it all the time, or only in the dead of night when you can't sleep, it's stress that in time will seem so normal you won't even notice it. That's when stress is at its most dangerous.

✧

WITH THE EXCEPTION OF incidents that arise suddenly—a car almost hitting us, a stranger lunging at us—fear usually arises when we project into the future. We ruminate on what might happen, what might go wrong. We imagine a future that isn't even remotely real, and then fear strides in and makes itself at home. Intellectually, we know that living in the present moment is a healthy thing to do. Eckhart Tolle's book *The Power of Now: A Guide to Spiritual Enlightenment* (2001) was a best seller and is still popular. Yet living right now, in this moment, is one of the hardest things to do. To some degree we obviously have to look ahead in life, and it can be productive to dream ahead—to visualize the future as we want it to be. But too often our travels outside the present moment result in what-if scenarios that scare us.

In dementia, all the person has is the present moment. Yes, they can wander into the past and often do, but they interpret even their past memories as occurring in the present. For example, a mother travels back in her mind to sixth grade when she shared her lunch with her best friend, Cheryl, because Cheryl never got anything good in her lunchbox. But this isn't experienced as a memory. In the mother's mind, she is there in the schoolyard with Cheryl. That is her present moment right then, until something else takes its place.

As difficult as it is to deal with, we can learn from this. In order to form any kind of bridge with someone who has dementia, we have to exist in the present moment with them, which activates some internal muscles that could use some stimulus. Standing still, confining ourselves to the moment at hand, takes discipline. Dealing with someone who has Alzheimer's, or any kind of dementia, is actually great training for how to live our lives.

❧

ONE DAY WHEN I went to my father's office to visit him, I arrived in the late morning, assuming he would be there. I knew his schedule. But I was told he was in the parking garage and there was a problem. I went to find him and he was in the back seat of the Secret Service car, very agitated, refusing to get out. I slid into the back seat beside him, and the two agents were doing their best to tell him it was okay to get out of the car, but he was having none of it. He was adamantly trying to tell us something, but his words were jumbled. What I got from him was fear, and that threw me. My father was a man who was never scared of anything. Seeing him look outside the car, motion to something he thought he was seeing, and show visible fear was something I had never experienced with him. I made a couple of feeble attempts to understand what he was saying, but it was clear that wasn't going to work. And then I thought, Okay, let's just stay with what's going on right now. He's scared of something outside this car. He was even putting a protective arm out across me, as he did when I was a kid and he had to suddenly hit the brakes.

One of the agents asked if they should just drive him home. That's when I thought, if something scares you, you get away from it. Immediately.

"Let's drive around the block," I said. "And then come back and see what happens."

As soon as we emerged into daylight and busy street traffic, my father's demeanor changed. Whatever was lurking in the shadows of the parking garage was gone, and so was his fear. I talked to him in soothing tones about nothing—the color of the car up ahead, a man crossing the street. I knew by then that the tone and cadence of my voice was the real communication. It took us about ten minutes to return to the garage, and he was fine. He got out of the car and went up to the office.

I had to get past my own trepidation to step into the moment and trust that if we changed the scenery, it might change my father's focus, and therefore his reality. These days, it's a commonly known tactic. Many of the techniques that are routinely used now with Alzheimer's patients became common knowledge because family members and hands-on caregivers figured them out.

Years ago, after giving a lecture for the opening of a new Memory Care facility, I was taken on a tour of the building. A doctor who worked at the facility was honest with me about how they designed and managed things there. He said so many decisions—from decorating the patients' rooms with personal items to making sure patients don't have to step from carpet to hard floor (which typically frightens Alzheimer's patients)—came from what family members told them. He said to me humbly, "As doctors we only see the patients sporadically. We don't see the patterns and the peculiarities of the disease the way family members do. So, we need to learn from the caregivers."

At this facility, they had re-created versions of the work that some of the residents once did. A lovely man with snow-white hair and blue eyes was walking around with a pile of manila folders and said as he passed that he was going to his office. I learned that he had been an optometrist, so they set up a small room for him with a chair facing a big eye chart on the wall, and the folders he was carrying were, in his mind, patient records. Another resident, a woman, used to be a seamstress, so they set her up in a room with a sewing machine (without a needle in it) and piles of fabric. These ideas came to them via family members.

✍

ONE OF THE THINGS that people dread the most with Alzheimer's is the inevitability of the person with the disease forgetting who their loved ones are. This isn't in the "if" column; it's in the "when" column, and everyone knows that. So, it builds up in people's minds as a huge marker. A common remark is, "When my mother forgets my name, then I'll think about getting full time care for her. But not until." Or "I don't know how I'll be able to visit with my father if he doesn't know who I am."

If you're willing to consider the premise I stated at the beginning of this book—that a person's soul can't be ill—then your loved one forgetting your name, or how you're related to them, is a malfunction in the circuitry of the brain. You live inside them on a deeper plane. Quite often, when people with Alzheimer's fail to recognize their children, or even their spouse, they mistake them for someone else, usually someone they care deeply for. So, a woman might look at her daughter and believe it's her sister, whom she loves. Both people take up room in her heart, both people stir up love in her; it's her brain that can't tell them apart.

There are, of course, instances of someone with dementia looking straight at a relative or spouse and reacting to them as if that person is a total stranger. It is unquestionably upsetting and painful, there is no getting away from that, but it's the brain that's misfiring, not the heart. If you hold onto that thought, it takes you out of the fear that bubbles up around this unrecognition. The real basis of the fear is the assumption that if your loved one doesn't recognize you, then they must no longer love you. But you don't know that's true; that's your interpretation. We need to take a wide view of what it is we are scared of. Once you identify the elements of your fear, it starts to diminish.

I suspected for a while that my father no longer knew who I was. Years into his illness, I was familiar to him—he knew my face and my voice, but I was pretty sure we had reached the point where he didn't know I was his daughter. In fact, there had been a couple of occasions when he said something about Patti, clearly not knowing that he was speaking to Patti. Something instinctual told me that these weren't isolated incidents; he really didn't know anymore who I was.

One afternoon, after I had visited with him for a while, I got up to leave and said, "'Bye Dad. I love you." His face softened into the most tender, appreciative smile, and he said, "Well, thank you. Thank you so much." It almost looked to me as if tears leaked into his eyes. To him, I was the nice woman who came and sat with him, was loving and kind to him, a woman he'd gone on walks with and watched sunsets with. He always brightened when I showed up. But because he didn't remember I was his daughter, hearing me say I loved him came as a surprise. This is how I chose to look at it: his response to a person he didn't know was related to him, who was telling him she loved him, was to be touched and grateful. It told me so much about the essence of who he was. He didn't recoil, he didn't bristle at such an intimate declaration—he sincerely said "Thank you." I have to admit that if a stranger came up to me and said, "I love you," I do not think I'd be so generous in my response.

☙

THERE IS MUCH TO be frightened of with dementia. I would never tell anyone to try to deny their fears. But fear becomes stress when it's left to fester in the dark. By dragging your fears out into the light, looking straight at them, you can diminish some of their power. If what you're scared of is not knowing what is coming next . . . guess what? None of us knows what's coming next in life, even when dementia isn't part of the story.

A friend of mine recently developed a mysterious skin condition. Her dermatologist told her it was probably "contact dermatitis," except she couldn't think of anything she'd come in contact with that was different or unusual. Then she began talking about the stress over her mother, who was showing cognitive decline as well as experiencing other health issues. My friend ended up describing perfectly what was going on with her own health. She said that on the surface she didn't appear to be stressed out, and in her daily life she didn't feel she was overly anxious. But underneath, she was raw with stress. I pointed out to her that she had just quite succinctly diagnosed the problem, and how logical it was that it would manifest as a skin condition. The stress was literally beneath her skin, and now it was working its way out. She has a very close relationship with her mother, and one of her biggest fears is having to say goodbye to her.

One of the best ways, I think, to disentangle ourselves from fear is to ask ourselves what is the worst that can happen. More often than not, in the context of dementia, our worst fear is that the person who is ill, the person we love, is going to die. When you haul that out into the light, you then have to acknowledge that, even without disease, death is moving closer simply because of their age. It's not going to hold off or disappear because you're afraid of it. So, given that it's inevitable, maybe a better course is to try to accept death as the closing of life's circle. Fear might still whisper into you, but it's less likely to paralyze you or cause physical ailments, because you've removed some of its power.

It's also possible to make friends with your fear if you have reverence for why it's there, if you're willing to examine it, look clearly at it, and occasionally even find humor in it. I remember someone saying to me that she was scared of the day when her mother would no longer know how to dress herself, until she realized she always hated the clothes her mother wore, so maybe it wouldn't be so bad if someone else dressed her.

✢

I MENTIONED THE VALUE of meditation earlier, but I want discuss it in more detail here. Meditation has been proven to lower anxiety and can therefore help prevent many of the health issues that caregivers are susceptible to, including depression. Yes, you are going to have to block out twenty or thirty minutes, and you will have to make sure that you aren't interrupted. This is one of the stumbling blocks—caregivers will say that it's impossible to take that time for themselves. But it isn't. Many have done it, many have found a way, and your health is worth it.

I think some of the resistance to meditation is the awareness that becoming quiet, going within, is going to unlock some feelings we've worked really hard to run away from. I've seen the wall come up in many people when I've suggested adding meditation to their daily schedule, and I've always tried to point out that emotions don't go away just because you bury them. In fact, it actually takes a lot of effort to bury them. So, you might as well sit quietly and see what comes up.

Many studies have been done on meditation and stress.[5] In fact, when I was running my support group at UCLA, several people in the group participated in a study on how meditation could help caregivers. It has been documented that meditation increases the protective tissues in the brain and reduces the stress hormone, cortisol. It also increases cortical thickness, which affects decision making and memory.

It doesn't matter what type of meditation you choose as long as you commit to doing it. You can find guided meditation, as well as other techniques, online. The point, obviously, is to slow down your brain, whichever method you choose. It's not easy. After many years I still have trouble on some days. But in the realm of caring for yourself, it's one of the best things you can do.

People caring for a loved one with dementia tend to think that the patient is the important one, and they themselves are not as important. Not only does that make no sense, it's a toxic attitude to have about yourself. Your health deserves attention too—both your physical health and your mental health. Everyone should remember that, no matter what their circumstances, but for caregivers, it's particularly important. It could keep you out of the hospital, or even save your life.

"Whatever you think you can do, or believe you can do, begin it. Action has magic, grace and power in it."

—GOETHE

CHAPTER 7

Creative Lying

As dementia progresses into what might be called the middle stages of the disease, reality—for the person with dementia—becomes a matter of opinion. It is not easy for a caregiver to deal with someone who insists the gardener is a spy or there is an antelope in the garage.

Most of us were raised with the instruction to always tell the truth. Lying was seen as something wrong, often a punishable offense. But in the world of Alzheimer's, lying is your friend. It's just another thing that this disease turns on its head. To tell someone with dementia the truth about why they can't go somewhere, or why they are wrong about what they're imagining to be true, is only going to stir up tension and angst. For example, if a relative is getting married, it could be a problem having a family member with dementia at the wedding, given the unpredictability of the disease. So, make something up. Tell your loved one that the couple is getting married underwater in scuba gear, or they're climbing to the top of a high mountain with only the chaplain. Lying in the service of kindness is not a punishable offense; in fact, I suspect it earns us karma points.

If your loved one thinks it's August and it's actually October, go with it. It doesn't matter. If they think their best friend from high school just came for a visit, ask how the visit went. The objective is to keep things peaceful. People with dementia may not be able to reason, but they definitely know when they are being contradicted.

I know someone whose close friend, a woman, has just been diagnosed with Lewy body dementia; along with two other friends, he has assumed many of the caregiving duties. Before they got her into the hospital to be diagnosed, she was having different sorts of delusions. One was that there were men on the roof. My friend tried to convince her that there were no men on the roof, that she was mistaken, and it erupted into an argument, with her insisting she saw the men. I suggested to him that, instead of telling her she was wrong, go outside, stay there for a few minutes, come back in and tell her that, yes, there were men on the roof, but they're gone now, and you don't think they'll be back. The goal is to keep things calm. That isn't achieved by arguing with someone who is certain that she saw men climbing on the roof. In her mind, she's right. Hallucinations are one of the symptoms of Lewy body dementia; this was very real to her. So, it was far better to play along, and tell her the intruders had left.

❧

ONE OF THE THINGS that happens as Alzheimer's progresses is "sundowning"[6]—meaning that as the day winds down, the person gets worse. Their cognition splinters more, they get increasingly confused. During one of these episodes, my father believed it was morning and he needed to go to the office. We told him that the office called and said he didn't need to come in because it was being fumigated, so no one was going to be allowed in. He accepted that, and shortly afterward forgot about going to the office.

On a sweeter note, my father once mentioned how he and I had gone ice-skating together when I was young. We never did. I remember going to an indoor rink when I was a child, but it was through a daytime summer camp and my father wasn't there. I caught myself just before I was about to correct him, and instead spun out an elaborate story about how we skated on a frozen pond, and he taught me how to skate backward. He was pulled into the story, followed every detail of what I was saying—how snow drifted down while we were skating and birds watched us from tree branches. When I left my parents' house that day I was overcome by a flood of tears, because I realized that I had duplicated what he used to do for me when I was very young. He created worlds with his stories, and I happily entered those worlds, never doubting for a second that they were real. Unicorns galloped through moonlight on cold winter nights; my goldfish that died was swimming in a wide blue river up in heaven, and no other fish would eat him because in heaven no one needed to eat. Now it was my turn to pull him into a world woven with my words. My childhood seemed far away, but the childlike way he listened to me brought it closer. The stories he once told me, so long ago, were of a gentler place, a place infused with magic. Near the end of his life, I had the chance to return that gift.

It is not easy to retrain yourself to tell lies. Think of it as an opportunity to stretch your creative muscles and exercise your imagination. Our instinct is to want to correct someone when they say something wrong, to set them straight on what the facts are. Early on in my father's illness, my mother told me that my father had been watching television and a football game was on. Suddenly, he got very agitated because he believed that this was his college football team and he was supposed to be there on the field. He thought he was late, he was letting them down, they needed him for the game. I think several people were trying to talk him down—my mother, a Secret Service agent, and a man who would come during the day to walk with my father and keep him company. His upset continued even after they turned the television off; he was definitely stuck in a loop, and I can't remember now how it ended. I think everyone, including my father, probably just got exhausted. But it spurred a conversation between me and my mother about the necessity of lying. Hearing about it long distance—I was still living in New York then—I could look at it through a calmer lens. We talked about how upsetting it is for anyone to hear that they are wrong, even someone with Alzheimer's. So, what if he were told that he hadn't been scheduled for that game? What if another player was getting his chance on the field, just for that one game? I remember my mother saying, "So, just lie to him?" To which I replied, "Why not?" I never heard of any other incidents quite like that again, so I assume she took the approach we discussed, although I also know that she told everyone to never again let him watch a football game on television.

IT's COMMON FOR PEOPLE with dementia to forget that relatives and friends have died. As they move backward through time, their parents and their friends who were with them in younger times are, to them, still alive. It's tempting to set the record straight and remind them that these people are gone, even to point out that they attended their funerals. The mistake there is that your loved one will have to mourn the loss all over again. And then they will probably forget again; if you keep reminding them it will be like some tear-stained version of *Groundhog Day*.

A member of my support group became very inventive with their parent, describing how the relatives who hadn't shown up for a visit were on a long ocean cruise, with no cellphone service. Time is a flexible thing with someone who has dementia, so this group member was able to spin out the story whenever the subject came up, adding colorful details and new destinations on this endless ocean cruise that deceased relatives were on. With Alzheimer's, every moment is new, so it always seemed like the first time the story was ever told. No detail was ever challenged or questioned.

One thing you can count on with Alzheimer's is that it will constantly change. If your loved one suddenly remembers that a relative or friend they were waiting for died years ago, go with it. Share in their memories of the loss, the aftermath, the funeral if there was one. And if a week later they are waiting for that same person to visit, having forgotten that they died, make something up for why they can't visit right then.

If you feel as though you are playing some crazy board game where the pieces are moving themselves, it's because you are. But you can guide things by coming up with stories designed to maintain some semblance of peace. You won't always be successful—upsets will happen. People with dementia can perseverate on something and it will seem they are never going to let it go. But they will. The bad thing about Alzheimer's is that people forget, and the good thing about Alzheimer's is that people forget. When someone is stuck in a loop, use your creativity—change the scenery, move them to a different room, take them for a walk, tell them a made-up story designed to capture their imagination. If the truth isn't going to be soothing, then tell a lie. A lie told from a place of kindness is, in the end, simply kindness. It's a small gesture in the whole scheme of things, but if you can avoid even a moment of upset, it matters.

"We know only too well that what we are doing is nothing more than a drop in the ocean. But if the drop were not there, the ocean would be different."   —MOTHER TERESA

CHAPTER 8

Anger

Many times someone in my support group would confess that they had gotten angry when their loved one was stuck in a loop, either behaviorally or verbally, and no amount of coaxing or distraction could resolve the situation. They felt awful that they had allowed their temper to flare, and they still felt guilty days later—long after their loved one had forgotten about it. One of my cofacilitators pointed out frequently that the anger was really directed at the disease, not the individual, even though that was how it was expressed in the moment. True, but anger can have different roots depending on a person's history.

Often someone who has a close, loving relationship with a parent who has dementia simply gets so exasperated that they lose their temper. Then they berate themselves because they feel they were unloving and insensitive. But their anger had nothing to do with their underlying emotions. Dealing with someone who has dementia is hard.

Hearing the same question thirty times over gets on your nerves. Listening to someone spin out a paranoid fantasy about men looking through the windows or people stealing from them during the night is bound to fray anyone's patience. In those situations, if you can remove yourself long enough to walk around the block or find someplace where you can growl and curse without being heard, do it. Give your anger an outlet other than directing it at your loved one.

The same applies to a spouse or partner, if that is the one with dementia. Unless there is some underlying issue in the relationship that predates the diagnosis, you aren't being unloving if anger gets the best of you in a particularly trying interlude. You're just being human.

It's a bit different if old resentments rise to the surface and manifest as anger. Like the man whose father hit him as a child, and constantly made him feel inferior. Now, that father can't remember how to tie his shoes, but he still remembers how to insult his son. Remember, Alzheimer's doesn't steal everything. Some patterns are deeply ingrained, so a parent who was abusive and demeaning is almost certainly not going to change his behavior. For the son to deal with his anger, he'll need more than a walk around the block. He'll need to thoroughly dissect that anger so he understands it, and then decide whether or not he wants to continue living with it.

There is a difference between *getting* angry and *being* angry. The latter—that state of being that is always simmering—is something I've had to address in my life.

As I've indicated, my mother was a very intimidating person, and I was always scared of her. At a fairly young age, I veered toward anger. It felt better than fear. That's the thing about anger—it always sits on top of something else, usually fear or grief. The adrenaline rush that we feel from anger is more palatable than the vulnerability that comes with being frightened or heartbroken. In fact, the adrenaline rush can feel good.

In the 1980s, when my father was president and I was voicing my disagreements a bit stridently at rallies and demonstrations, I was at the airport one day when a slender white-haired woman recognized me. "You're a very angry person," she said, and then walked away.

Something inside me froze. I knew she was right, but I didn't know what to do about it. I think I assumed it was something that had imprinted me so long ago that I would never be rid of it. It took me many years, a lot of therapy, and a lot of work to realize that no emotion is permanent. We can overcome anything, but we have to be willing to take it apart and look at all the components. I finally figured out that anger was, to a large extent, my substitute for emotions I didn't want to deal with.

Dementia is tricky for the caregiver when it comes to defining the cause of his or her own emotions. It's easy to say, "I'm just angry because of this unfair disease." Or "I just lose my temper when my parent becomes irascible and obstinate." And sometimes, for some people, that's true. But there are other situations in which a lifetime of emotions comes into play. I think we are all more aware of our internal landscapes than we like to admit. When there is old, timeworn anger in you, you know it.

Dementia provides you with an opportunity to change something you've spent years turning away from. It's a choice, though—you can keep turning away from it, but then you'll miss learning the valuable lessons that dementia can teach.

By now, I've heard many stories of abuse and neglect by a parent who, decades later, is diagnosed with some form of dementia. I would never try to minimize the pain that a son or daughter experienced, nor would I ever suggest that their wounds aren't valid and their anger isn't justified. What I have tried to communicate, what I hope to get across here, is that living with that kind of anger isn't serving anyone well.

One winter morning, when I was still living in New York, I walked across Central Park to Wolman Rink to go ice-skating. A small group of people would go early, before the rink opened to the public, so it had just gotten light when I set out. It was drizzly, and there was a forecast of rain; I was told the rink would only be open for a little while. As soon as the ice started to get too wet, it was going to close. No one else was there. I went out on the ice alone in the gray damp air, the city rumbling around me, and my thoughts turned to a dream I'd had the night before that was troubled and turbulent. I was a child in the dream, and my mother was in it, but beyond that I couldn't remember much, except that I was so overcome with both fear and anger that when I woke up my heart was racing.

As I skated around, I let myself linger on the slivers of the dream that I could recall, and something came to me. I suddenly felt gratitude for my anger; I realized that it had kept me from being pulled under by my fear. I saw that for decades it had been my lifeline. Without it, I would almost surely have been overwhelmed by the feelings I wasn't yet equipped to deal with. Seeing it through that lens changed everything for me and helped me recognize that I didn't need that anger anymore. In fact, to keep holding onto it meant I was giving my past an awful lot of power.

❧

IT'S NOT EASY TO let go of emotions you have relied on for a long time. I picture it like this: It's as if you've been in rough waters, holding onto a rope for years because without it, you know you'll drown. Then someone comes along and says, "It's okay, you can let go. You actually can swim just fine." Your first reaction will be, "Oh no, I don't think so. I think I should keep holding on. It's worked for me for years." Then you let the idea of swimming free settle in and some part of you decides to give it a try. It was a good strong rope to hang onto, and you should thank it for its service, but you don't need it anymore.

Of course, once you let go of the rope, you have to deal with the waters around you. It was startling for me to have to admit to myself how huge my fear of my mother was. Many times I wanted to bounce back into anger—it felt like an easier place to be. But I thought about my father and the disease that was whittling him away; I thought about time and how I didn't know how much of it we had left. I didn't want to spend that remaining time with the same level of anger I had carried around with me for so many years. It's hard for any of us to see beyond anger, and there was so much I wanted to see.

Moments come, in the progression of Alzheimer's, when you get a new glimpse into your loved one, whether it's a parent or spouse or sibling. Those moments are gone in the blink of an eye. If fragments of the past, especially your resentments, are in the way, you'll miss them. A man told me that his mother, who was deep into Alzheimer's, had been cruel to him as a child, even beating him at times. He had decided at a certain point to forgive her so that he could move on with his life. He would always have the memories of a traumatic childhood, but he didn't want to live anymore with the emotional wreckage she had caused. One day when he was visiting her, her eyes focused on him and there was something present and deliberate in her look, which made him pay close attention. Suddenly, in almost a whisper, she said, "I'm sorry." He carried those two words with him in his heart like a talisman. He hadn't asked for them, he hadn't expected them, but he knew that if he hadn't cleared his own internal vision by forgiving his mother, he either would have missed that moment, or he would have dismissed it as meaningless—just words uttered with nothing behind them. Instead, he believed her words meant exactly what he hoped they meant.

As cognition becomes more fragmented in someone with dementia, their emotions become more present; so does their awareness of other people's emotions. If you're angry around your loved one, he or she no longer has the cognitive ability to understand where your anger is coming from, so there is no rational thought to act as a buffer. All they experience is a tide of emotion coming at them. And if you think you're concealing your anger, you should probably think again. We are all more transparent than we assume we are. That's why the woman at the airport could so confidently tell me what an angry person I was. Our thoughts, our emotions, resonate with others even if we think we're being subtle and hiding them. We communicate with each other on many levels; language is just one of them. Our thoughts and feelings travel between us on a mysterious plane. And just because someone has dementia, it doesn't mean they don't pick up on those thoughts and feelings.

Ken Keyes's book *The Hundredth Monkey* illustrated the power of the collective unconscious.[7] In 1952 some scientists went to the Japanese island of Kojima to study the macaque monkeys who lived there. They watched as the older monkeys washed the sweet potatoes that were their main food source before eating them. Then they observed the younger monkeys imitating their elders; they also started to wash the sweet potatoes before eating them. When it got to the hundredth monkey, all the monkeys on the island began washing their food. Then they discovered that on all the surrounding islands, monkeys had suddenly begun washing their food before they ate it.

Whether or not you believe the story in its entirety (and there has been some controversy over it), it is meant to illustrate the power of thought and how it can transcend language and intentional communication, how it can travel on an invisible plane. That linkage of thoughts and emotions doesn't fall apart because someone has dementia. It functions on an intuitive plane that's different from basic cognition.

While dealing with your own deep emotions can definitely have a beneficial effect on a loved one who has dementia, it's not just about them. It's about you and the path of your life. We all have broken places in us; we all have been wounded in some way and we have the scars to prove it. For many people, those broken places happened in childhood, at the hands of a parent. The truth is that those broken places will always be there. You will always have the history you had; you can't go back and change it or even heal it. What you can do is build up some emotional musculature around the weak places so they don't define you. I've heard people talk about the families they have created with close friends where they have found the love and support that wasn't there with their biological family. I've also heard people say that getting involved with charity work gave them the sustenance and self-worth they didn't get when they were growing up.

A long time ago I knew a man who had injured his knee numerous times playing sports. This was long before knee-replacement surgery was available, so there weren't many options for him. He trained and worked out religiously, and he told me that he had built up his leg muscles so that they were literally holding his knee in place. I think that's a great metaphor for what we need to do emotionally.

Rather than think, "How do I take away these wounds?" or "How do I undo the damage my abusive parent caused?" think about adding things internally that will strengthen and develop your emotional musculature, so that those broken places, those old wounds, are just a small part of you. They represent things that happened to you, they do not represent who you are.

✽

PEOPLE WITH DEMENTIA ARE imprisoned in their past. They will move back through time, they will revisit periods of their life, and nothing you do or say can change that. They don't have the option of choosing to interpret their experiences differently or working to look at their history through a different lens. If they were a negligent or cruel parent, that will remain their prison. But you don't have to be imprisoned by their past. To not accept the invitation that Alzheimer's is offering—namely to get rid of old paradigms—is to keep giving power to a person you have resented for years.

People often say, "Well, I need to feel what I'm feeling." That is absolutely true. I would never advise anyone to deny the anger that they feel. But there is a difference between feeling an emotion and living inside of it for protracted periods of time.

It has been interesting, in the long siege of the coronavirus pandemic, to see how our collective anger has escalated. At first, people were generally concerned for one another. There was a sense of connection, of shared hardship, a camaraderie even among strangers. We all grieved over the loss of normal life, which had been so abruptly snatched away from us. But as months rolled on, the grief deepened. Deaths kept mounting and people couldn't be with their loved ones at the end; too many people lost jobs, income, health insurance. It's almost as if the grief became too much to bear, so anger took over. Why so much of that anger centered on the necessity of wearing masks is completely irrational, but anger needs a focal point. Collectively right now, at the time of writing, anger is sitting on top of the grief and fear that we all feel—fear of getting the virus, fear of losing homes and livelihoods. I've certainly felt in myself the temptation to get angry rather than to own how sad and terrifying this time in the world is.

In the realm of dementia, whether you get angry at a loved one in a moment of exasperation or your history with that person is stoking your anger, ask yourself the same question: is this really where I want to be? Hopefully, the answer is no. A pretty effective technique is to set a time limit on your anger. Thirty minutes, one hour—during that time you can feel as angry as you want (not, of course, at another person). Find a physical outlet: hit a punching bag, go for a run, stew over whatever is making you mad, grind your teeth, practice swear words . . . but when the time is up, stop. You don't get extra time. Frequently giving yourself an hour to be completely furious will lead you to get tired of your own anger after about forty-five minutes.

None of us is going to avoid anger entirely, not in our daily lives and certainly not in the trying situation of being a caregiver for someone with dementia. The best we can do is figure out ways to manage it, to keep it in its place so it doesn't come to define who we are.

"All the art of living lies in a fine mingling of letting go and holding on."
—HAVELOCK ELLIS

CHAPTER 9

Guilt and the Balm of Laughter

When I first learned of my father's diagnosis, I was acutely aware of the guilt that found its way into my thinking. How would I atone for my past sins, the times I had hurt him and disregarded his feelings, if Alzheimer's was stealing him away? How would I reach across an impossible chasm created by a disease I didn't even understand? There were, in the early days and months, quiet times when I joined him for a walk or sat with him in a slant of afternoon sunlight, when I spoke to him about my regrets—how I wished I had expressed myself differently in the turbulence of the eighties, when I publicly and stridently opposed his policies. I should have listened more in those years even if I didn't agree with him. I was disrespectful back then and I carried the burden of remorse. Sometimes he nodded and said a few words of acknowledgment, sometimes he said nothing and just fixed his eyes on me, but I believed then and believe now that he heard me, deep in his soul. Just as I felt guilt push its way in, I felt it drift away.

Which doesn't mean I was done with guilt. Alzheimer's doesn't let you off that easily. Years later, in my support group, I would hear other people express the same feelings I had experienced—the pressure when they couldn't understand what their loved one was trying to say, or when things that had happened in the past nudged them from behind. We end up berating ourselves because we feel we could have done better. We could have fixed things. Wanting to fix things is where much of the problem exists.

We're accustomed to a world in which there is a solution for every dilemma. If we can't find it ourselves, we call someone who will diagnose the problem and remedy it. But Alzheimer's is a different world. There is no fixing the disease or the various problems that it engenders. There are techniques for managing certain situations, but no guarantee that these will fix the difficulty at hand. If they don't work, too often our own guilt grabs hold of us and says, "What's wrong with you? You should have been able to deal with this."

Once when I was at my parents' house my father got it in his head that he was wearing contact lenses, which he had worn for more than half his life but wasn't doing anymore, since expecting someone with Alzheimer's to manage contact lenses is inadvisable. He was pinching his eyeballs, trying to remove lenses that weren't there. No one could convince him that he didn't have contacts in his eyes, and I feared he was going to injure himself. I asked him to look in my eyes to see the lenses I was wearing, and then compare that to his eyes, where no lenses were visible. It didn't work. I felt I should be the one to fix this, simply because I was the only one there who wore contact lenses. I led him outside and asked him to look at the view from his hillside home. I held his eyeglasses in my hand. He looked out, squinted, and seemed confused; then I handed him his glasses. "See how clear things are with your glasses?" I said to him. "If you had contacts in, you wouldn't need your glasses. But without your glasses everything is blurry."

I'm not sure if it was the initial blurriness of the view, or just walking him outside, that worked. I felt guilty afterward for not being able to fix the situation right away. It was illogical, but I couldn't seem to shake myself out of it.

That day stayed with me for a while. I would wonder what I could do if he and I were going for a walk and he got it in his head that he had contact lenses in that needed to come out. When I was growing up, my father had a habit of taking a contact lens out, putting it in his mouth to wet it or clean it, and then replacing it in his eye. He'd even do it at red lights when he was driving the station wagon home from the ranch. It was an unsanitary habit and my brother Michael and I adopted it until we knew better. So I knew how deeply rooted the memory of wearing contacts was in my father, and I felt burdened with the responsibility of dealing with it if it came up again.

Finally, exhausted by the pressure I was putting on myself, I came up with this: Guilt is like a muscle that needs to flex itself sometimes. Sort of like fear—we need it, just not all the time. It's good that we have that guilt muscle; if we didn't, we could do horrible things and never feel any remorse. So, I didn't want to remove guilt completely from my life, I just wanted it not to activate itself at inappropriate times. I decided to have an internal dialogue with it. The next time my father said something I couldn't make sense of, I said to my guilt: "I'm glad you're here, you're very important, but I don't need you right now." It sounds silly, and that's part of the point. It took me out of the cycle of self-punishment, which can get too serious too quickly and become relentless.

One of the triggers for guilt, in the strange and off-kilter world of dementia, is humor. Dementia can be such a bleak landscape that caregivers often feel as though there is no room for laughter or lightness. One of the things I treasured in my support group was that we laughed a lot. There were plenty of tears as well, but humor was a balm to the pain that everyone was experiencing. We weren't laughing *at* anyone, we were simply laughing because there are things in the world of Alzheimer's that are funny. People with dementia sometimes say funny things; often the predicaments that come up, while not amusing at the time, in hindsight can be looked at with humor, and there is a catharsis to that.

Someone told me a story about a plane trip they took with their mother who had Alzheimer's; she should not have been flying, but the family didn't realize that at the time. Midway into the flight, the woman got extremely upset and no one could calm her down. She climbed over seats, trying to get into the cockpit, yelling at passengers. In fact, I think she actually did open the door to the cockpit. (This was before 9/11; if it had been after, they'd have landed the plane on the nearest runway and removed her.) The person who was recounting this told it in such a funny way, with so much detail, that we both laughed. Then they suddenly stopped and said, "I shouldn't be making light of this. It was horrible." I could see guilt wash over them. I pointed out that, of course it was awful when it was happening; fortunately, no one was hurt in all the chaos. But there is no reason to not find humor in it now. Neither of us was laughing out of cruelty, or hard-heartedness. We were simply laughing because the visual recollection of the incident was funny. And, more important, because the person who went through it, who was telling the story, needed that laughter.

If you question how important laughter is to your health, read Norman Cousins's book *Anatomy of an Illness*.[8] Cousins was diagnosed with an almost-always-fatal degenerative disease, and he cured himself—to the surprise of doctors—with a deliberately crafted program of laughter as well as massive injections of Vitamin C. He details in the book how different he felt after watching a funny movie and laughing uproariously—how he could sleep peacefully with less pain and discomfort. I had the immense pleasure of getting to know Cousins a bit in the mid-eighties. He came to my wedding. I will always treasure what I learned from him, and I will always wonder if I could have learned more. He was one of those people who, it seemed, would always be here. There are moments when I'm haunted by the thought that I might not have taken full advantage of our brief friendship.

Once when we were talking, Norman said, "Laughter is inner jogging." In the stress of being a caregiver, laughter can be one of your lifelines. Emotionally, psychologically, and even physically, you need it. An added benefit is that it can be infectious. Someone with dementia is still affected by others laughing around them and often wants to join in; the disease doesn't take that away. And it doesn't matter if they understand why they're laughing, it just matters that they are.

At times my father would make a goofy face or have a silly reaction to something, and we would laugh simply because it was funny. In that moment, Alzheimer's was pushed to the side—we'd have laughed just the same under normal circumstances. His face would light up, he'd start laughing too, and then do something else to continue the levity—another silly face or gesture. There is a misguided notion that we're being somehow disloyal to the gravity of Alzheimer's by finding moments of humor. But by not finding humor, by not laughing, we're letting the darkest parts of the disease win.

✑

OCCASIONALLY IN MY support group people would mention that they had read about some experimental remedy for Alzheimer's, like a diet of coconut oil, and they would feel guilty that they weren't trying it. One person read a story about a very wealthy man who had traveled the country taking his wife to every healer, doctor, or pseudo-doctor who promised a potential cure for the disease. This group member felt guilty about not spending exorbitant amounts of money doing the same thing. The only way to dismantle that kind of emotional assault is to use logic.

So far, no one has been able to stop the progression of Alzheimer's once it has claimed its victim. And as far as spending vast amounts of money on experimental treatments and possible cures, wouldn't that money be better spent on care for the loved one who is ill? The wealthy man in that news story (which I had read, too) certainly wasn't going to be destitute after spending so much. And he had every right to pursue whatever he thought might help. But it was still futile, and while I respect his intentions and his doggedness, I wish someone had talked him out of it. Not because of the money, but because of the exhausting cycle of hope and disappointment. He wasn't only wearing himself down, he was putting his wife through unnecessary ordeals.

Some of the bravest people I've ever met are those who have taken on the task of being a caregiver, in whatever way they have.

People who came to the support group looking for help, searching for answers and sustenance, who were willing to change their thinking and open their hearts, had nothing to feel guilty about. Theirs was a quiet, persistent courage that endured through the ragged days and dark nights of a ruthless disease. Guilt has no place there. It broke my heart to hear people berating themselves for imagined faults when all I saw was astounding courage.

AN AREA IN WHICH guilt can arise with a vengeance is relationships with siblings. I mentioned earlier that it's rare to find a family that is bonded and cohesive in its approach to a parent diagnosed with dementia. In six years of running Beyond Alzheimer's, I can only think of a few examples when that was the case. Typically, in most families, one offspring takes the helm. This can be because he or she has been chosen by the parent, it can be because the other siblings don't want the responsibility, or it can be a sort of power-grab that has left everyone else in the dust. What's always clear is that the dynamic between siblings was forged long before dementia entered the picture; it just becomes more dramatic and more obvious in the context of illness.

So, a son who has been sidelined by a bossy sister can end up feeling guilty that he isn't doing more to help the parent who has dementia. But every time he tries to intervene—suggest something or change the way things are being handled—she shuts him down. Inevitably, arguments arise that then lead to more guilt. Or there can be the opposite situation, in which one sibling takes on the burden of responsibility because the others don't want to, and then feels guilty because his or her parent keeps asking where the others are.

Family complications don't fade when dementia enters the picture; they get worse because they're being dragged out into the light. In almost every case, what you are going through now is just another version of what you've always gone through. If there are moments when your siblings might be open to looking at the history you share, and seeing how patterns are repeating themselves, seize those moments. It's not impossible that things can change, but it's going to take everyone being on board for that. You didn't create the situation all by yourself, and you can't remedy it all by yourself.

My family was always fractured and distant, with each person traveling in his or her own lane of life, so no one expected that we would come together and have deep discussions about what was happening to our father. One evening in my support group, when I was listening to someone describe a volatile situation among siblings, with arguments and disagreements, I found myself feeling strangely envious. In my family, none of the siblings knew each other that well; distance whistled between us, and other than on holidays like Christmas we rarely saw each other. We weren't close enough to argue. It struck me that there is an intimacy and a closeness to that kind of messiness—to arguing and disagreeing; maybe looking at it that way could be a valuable perspective. If the alternative is not knowing your brothers and sisters well at all, arguing doesn't seem like such a bad thing. At least you're communicating.

In the early years of my father's Alzheimer's, my half sister Maureen and I made a valiant attempt to get to know each other. She was going through treatment for melanoma and was basically housebound in Los Angeles, and I was still living in New York, so we had many long-distance calls. I remember the awkwardness of wondering how this sister thing is supposed to work. It was like a foreign language to both of us, but we forged ahead. I remember one call in early November. She was feeling stronger, and I was going to fly back to California soon, so we planned to see each other. She asked me if I was staying for Thanksgiving, and I told her that my mother had stopped celebrating Thanksgiving a couple of years earlier. She had simply announced, "We don't do Thanksgiving anymore," which seemed sadly appropriate since Thanksgiving is the ultimate family occasion and we were a family that didn't know how to be one.

Maureen desperately wanted to have Thanksgiving with our father. She asked me to try to convince my mother to change her mind, even saying that she would do most of the cooking. I tried, but I hit a wall. It just wasn't going to happen. I felt horribly guilty that I couldn't give Maureen what she wanted, what would have meant so much to her. But then I had to remind myself that this was the reality of our family. I couldn't change it by myself, and neither could Maureen. I wrestled myself out of guilt's unpleasant grip and accepted that in this regard my family was not going to change.

℘

YOU CAN'T REALLY AVOID your family members, but you can be discerning about the friends and acquaintances you let in. Some will have opinions about how an Alzheimer's patient should be treated, about the choices that caregivers and family members should make. Even if they mean well, it's really none of their business. Find the people who will support you, who will listen and not intrude in a way that makes you feel uncomfortable or suggest you are doing things wrong or not doing enough.

Shortly after I moved back to California I ran into a woman I had known when I was married. She was a friend of my husband's, and I had never particularly liked her, mostly because she made it clear she didn't like me. But there she was, so I was polite. She then launched into a sales pitch for some healer she knew who, she believed, could cure Alzheimer's.

"He doesn't see that many people," she said, with an air of haughtiness. "But if you use my name, he'd probably see you. He's very expensive, but he might give you a break on his fee since I recommended you."

I won't go into the responses that ran through my head—just use your imagination. Restraining myself, I said to her, "Thank you, but I think we're beyond anything like that."

"Well," she huffed. "If it were my father, I'd want to do whatever I could to help him."

As angry as I was at her insensitivity and rudeness, I still felt the grip of guilt when she accused me of not wanting to help my father. I have heard similar versions of this from other people—conversations in which friends or acquaintances insist that they know best what should be done when it comes to another person's loved one. If it's a friend you care about and want in your life, tell them that you appreciate their concern but that if you want their suggestions you will ask for them. If the friend doesn't listen and continues to intrude, you might have to make a hard decision about whether or not this person should remain in your life. Being a caregiver for a loved one with dementia is hard enough without people who don't know the intricacies and inner workings of your family weighing in on what they think you should be doing.

※

ONE OF THE COFACILITATORS in my support group said often that the antidote for guilt is gratitude. I loved that idea the moment I heard it. It can be a bit jarring at first for caregivers who are dealing with dementia to hear about gratitude. But even in the midst of grief and loss, even when a disease like Alzheimer's dominates a family's life, there are still things to be grateful for.

I mentioned earlier that the "long goodbye" of Alzheimer's can be looked at as a gift when compared to sudden and brutal deaths in mass shootings or other tragedies. Time, as it stretches out and seems to slow down, is a gift to treasure. Dementia is not a disease of wrenching physical pain. The suffering that dementia patients might experience when drifting back through the years and landing on certain memories can be hard to watch, but it's short-lived. They will move on; they will forget what upset them. That too is something to acknowledge and feel grateful for.

When I think back on my father's illness, what comes to me first are the moments that shine brightly out of the shadows of Alzheimer's. I think of the afternoon when a rainstorm had just ended and I was sitting outside with him at my parents' house. The view was sparkling and clean. The billowing clouds overhead, the trees, and the city in the distance looked like a painting. He turned to me and said, "He does good work." I wasn't sure what he meant, but I guessed. "God?" I asked him. "Yep," he answered, his eyes twinkling as they used to many years before.

I think of walking with him along the boardwalk at the beach and the way he gazed out at the ocean. I wondered if he was longing to run across the sand and plunge into the waves the way he once could. There was something in his eyes that looked like a mix of loss and longing. People passing by would recognize him and call out greetings, almost always addressing him as either Mr. President or President Reagan. He'd always wave back and say hello to them. One day he turned to me and said, "They all seem to know me. How do they know me?" I explained that they recognized him because he was famous when he was president of the United States years ago. He looked bewildered, shook his head a little like he was trying to jar a memory into place. But it didn't work. He didn't remember. I wanted to change the look in his eyes, so I started talking to him about the ocean. "Nothing to be scared of with the ocean," he said. And there was no fear in his eyes, no bewilderment, just the memory of water and tides.

I think about the Christmas when our whole family was together, when my father looked at the tree and asked, "Why is there a tree in here?" Michael tried explaining to him that it was Christmas, and this was the Christmas tree. It didn't register. I recall that a few of us tried to explain the holiday, with no luck. It finally became clear that the concept of Christmas was not registering. He was asking a very basic question: Why is there a tree in the living room? Eventually, we figured out that the key was just to answer the question simply. We told him that at this time of year, everyone puts pine trees in their living rooms, and we were just doing what everyone else was doing. He seemed to mull it over, nodded, and then said emphatically, "Okay. Well, there you go." It sticks out in my mind because he showed us something about dealing with Alzheimer's—sometimes you just need to answer the specific question in the most basic way, without inserting concepts like holidays or special occasions.

I think about the day I went on a walk with him at a park near my parents' house. We were on a sidewalk across the street from the park when, from behind a gate, a dog barked at us. My father turned and barked back at the dog. At first, I was embarrassed. I looked around to see if anyone was nearby other than his Secret Service agents. I didn't want someone to see Ronald Reagan barking at a dog. But then my father looked at me and laughed. I thought, "Who cares if someone sees him? The world knows he has Alzheimer's, and he's having a good time."

I think of all these moments and more with immense gratitude. Putting guilt in its place, asking it to leave the premises when it's not needed, is a process that is ongoing. Even when I knew better, I felt guilty sometimes—when I laughed with my father, when I felt a sense of peace unexpectedly wash over me, it would seem for a moment as if I were being disloyal to the seriousness of the disease. I had to remind myself again and again that there are many colors on the palette of Alzheimer's—some dark, some brighter. I owed it to myself, and I owed it to my father, to embrace all of them. Gratitude was one of the brightest colors, and it has followed me through the years, anchoring my memories and reminding me that as complicated as life can be, it can also be as simple as a shiny afternoon after the rain has passed and it feels like God is smiling.

"The deeper that sorrow carves into your being, the more joy you can contain."   —KHALIL GIBRAN, "On Joy and Sorrow"

CHAPTER 10

Losing a Life Partner

It's heartbreak that no one is prepared for. When one's spouse or partner is diagnosed with dementia, the despair is so deep, the loneliness so crippling, it seems as though the earth has shifted on its axis. When we commit to another person, we know that if fate so determines, he or she might die before us. But no one is prepared for a partner to leave while still there physically. No one can foresee how vast the emptiness can be when the person next to you, with whom you have shared years, is out of reach. You know every inch of their body, you know the rise and fall of their breath as they sleep, the sound of their footsteps on the floor, the touch of their hand on your face. And all of that is there, right beside you, but who they have always been is a million miles away. Time becomes the enemy; every day, every week, they move farther away. Memories turn punishing, since they now belong only to you. While there are, of course, similarities to losing a parent to dementia, the wound of losing a spouse cuts deeper into the heart, and people are more reluctant to talk about it.

My father was a few months away from the end of his life when, as I was leaving my parents' house one day, my mother collapsed against me. Sobbing, she said, "Nothing will ever be the same without him." I put my arms around her and tried to comfort her. This was completely unfamiliar. I didn't know the feel of my mother's embrace. I had seen it in home movies when I was young, so I knew there were times when she wrapped her arms tightly around me, but I had no memory of it, and somewhere along the line she felt disinclined toward that kind of affection. So, conversely, I had never embraced her, at least not in the years beyond childhood.

It was midafternoon. Pale light spilled through the tall glass windows and drifted across the floor of the entryway where we stood. Her tears soaked through my shirt onto my skin. A lifetime stood between us. To my right hung the Norman Rockwell painting of my father—several images of his face, his blue eyes bright and blazing. Down the hall, in the room where he lay in a hospital bed, his eyes were closed much of the time, and when they were open, they weren't that blue anymore. I kept urging my heart to memorize the painting.

Almost ten years had passed from the time when he wrote a letter that began with "My fellow Americans, I have recently been told that I am one of the millions of Americans who will be afflicted with Alzheimer's disease." He ended the letter by saying, "I now begin the journey that will take me into the sunset of my life." During the years that followed, I started to look at my parents' relationship through a softer lens. For most of my life, I'd harbored some resentment for the exclusionary nature of their bond. They formed a complete circle, with everyone else, even their children, orbiting outside of it. But as

Alzheimer's shattered their once-secure world, I saw that there was a cost to having lived in a world of two. My mother had no idea how to let anyone in to comfort her—not her children, not anyone.

Early in the disease, I noticed that my mother was still asking my father questions. It was clear that he seemed confused much of the time, and didn't know how to answer her, especially if she began a question with, "Honey, do you remember . . . ?" At first, I found myself annoyed. Didn't she see that this was not a good idea? But then I realized that she didn't know how to behave any differently with my father. This was how they had communicated for decades. I saw so clearly her loneliness. I saw her reaching out for contact with him, for communication, for the once-easy sharing that was now gone. I realized that losing my father was, for her, like losing an appendage. She would have to learn how to function in an entirely new way.

The wound of losing your partner to dementia is deep whether you have been together for five years or fifty years, whether the situation is early-onset Alzheimer's or dementia that strikes later in life. But I think there are more complications when a couple has been together for many decades, winding around each other like tree roots, getting sustenance from one another for so long it's inconceivable that they will have to exist apart.

In a rare moment of vulnerability, my mother admitted to me that she often chattered away at my father, knowing he wouldn't respond, because she was overwhelmed with loneliness. For that same reason, she said, she kept the television on for hours every day—to fill the house with the sound of people talking. "It makes me feel less alone," she said. Once I carefully suggested that asking him questions might not be such a good idea. She said, "I know. I just don't know how else to talk to him."

Sporadically, throughout my father's illness, my mother would do interviews with Larry King on his talk show. On one of her appearances, when he was asking about the emotional toll Alzheimer's was taking on her, she replied that it was terribly hard, but she had a network of friends who were there for her. She said nothing about family members. I might have been hurt by that, but the exclusion was familiar. By then, it was old news to me. So, instead of checking myself to see if she had drawn blood, I thought about how sad it was for her that she had never brought her children and stepchildren into her world, so that when hard times came there would be a family unit that could easily and naturally fall into place around her pain. As lonely as this disease is, having family around to absorb some of the pain can make a huge difference. I witnessed times when my half brother Michael tried to get past my mother's long-standing resentment of him to comfort her, and she would have none of it. I don't think she ever realized what she lost by pushing us away.

Watching one parent being conquered by dementia and the other consumed by loss can be frustrating and depressing. It can seem as though nothing you do for the parent who is the caregiver is enough. If you are in that situation, know that your presence and your support matter. You fill up some of the loneliness, you soothe the edges of his or her sadness, even if you can't abolish it entirely. The caregiver parent might be too overwhelmed to tell you that you're making a difference, but know that you are. This is a passage of your parents' relationship that they have to navigate themselves. You can be there, you can offer comfort, but the caregiver is going to have to find his or her way through it.

A man I met at a lecture I gave years ago made a courageous admission to me. His wife of forty-four years was deep into Alzheimer's; she had round-the-clock care at that point. He told me that, even though it wasn't rational or logical, a part of him was angry at her for leaving him in this way—stolen by such a cruel disease. He said that they had, many years earlier, discussed death, and what their end-of-life wishes were; they had drawn up the proper documents. He had imagined her death preceding his. He had never imagined her abandoning him like this—absent while she was still there physically—and it made him angry. He quickly emphasized that he knew it wasn't her fault: he wasn't blaming her, but he was acutely aware of the feelings that rose up in him. It illuminated for me the fact that there is much to be angry about with this disease, and if we can be open enough to talk about the emotions that arise, we have a better chance of moving through them.

I will never know all the emotions that washed down on my mother, that kept her awake in the dead of night—our relationship didn't allow for such sharing of confidences. But those who do have a close relationship with their parents can learn a lot about them in the difficult years of dementia. Typically, none of us think about our parents in any way except as our parents. We conveniently forget that they had a life together before they were our parents. But the caregiver who is living through the slow loss of his or her life partner might want to share their inner struggles as the disease progresses, so it's important to be alert to those signs. Even if they don't, by just paying attention you might be able to see things about your parents that you never observed before.

What you're noticing is not just about them, it's about all of us—our frailties and strengths as human beings. The point of looking through different eyes is to get a wider view. When I look at my parents in our home movies—a young couple with their chubby new baby—I'm seeing them through different eyes. I'm not trapped in the narrow space of who they were as my parents. That helped me as the end moved closer because I could look at my mother as a woman going through the wrenching pain of losing her soulmate, and none of my history with her intruded on my compassion.

Frequently in my support group people brought up things they had noticed in their parents' relationship after one parent had been diagnosed with dementia. Usually, it was a pattern or habit of behaving that had always been there but suddenly seemed problematic given the family's new reality. It could be anything from mild bickering to bossiness or nagging. In the heightened atmosphere of Alzheimer's, things that once seemed normal can now appear alarming. Taking a step back and looking at things differently is really important at this time. If this is how your parents have always been with each other, this is home to them. Obviously, if something like bickering gets worse and accelerates, or turns abusive, that needs to be addressed. But if your parents are just behaving the way they always did, they're fine. Those familiar roles are comfortable for them. There will come a point when things change, just as my mother had to realize she couldn't talk to my father in the same way anymore. She couldn't reminisce with him, she couldn't ask him questions. It was wrenching for her, and sad to watch.

This chapter of your parents' lives is not their whole story. It's not your whole story either. It's what life has brought you to now, and when it ends—which it will—there is an opportunity to infuse the rest of your days with lessons you learned. I'm still discovering things that I learned from my father's Alzheimer's. But one thing I'm clear about is that everything I learned came from constantly reminding myself to look at things from different angles.

A SHORT WHILE AFTER my father needed to be in a hospital bed, my mother said she couldn't sleep in their king-size bed anymore. The space around her was too vast without him there beside her, on his side of the bed. She had the bed removed and got a queen-size bed, but instead of buying new sheets, she had the king-size sheets taken to a seamstress and cut down. I pointed out that it would probably cost her a lot less to just buy new queen-size sheets, but she jutted out her chin, gave me one of her looks, and said, "I like those sheets. Your father and I slept on those sheets for years." I backed off.

I found it fascinating that she wanted their bed out of there, but she had to have something familiar to hang onto. When the new bed was brought in, there was a visible mark on the carpet where the old bed had been for years. The rest of the carpet in the room had faded, but the part that had been beneath the bed was a couple of shades darker. It was quite noticeable. I waited to see if she was going to say something about it—maybe have the entire carpet replaced—but she never did. In time, the dark patch faded as well. But for many months, whenever I went into her room, I thought of it as a ghost of the part of their relationship that had been stolen from them. My father breathed on the other side of the wall now, in a different room, in a hospital bed that was adjusted frequently so he wouldn't get bedsores. He was watched by nurses who tended to him day and night, but if he had dreams, he couldn't roll over and tell my mother about them. I don't know if it helped her to get a smaller bed, if it eased any of her loneliness. I think she just felt she had to change something. Until the end of her life, she still slept on "her" side of the bed.

BY WATCHING MY PARENTS' relationship as Alzheimer's moved in so relentlessly, and in listening to the stories of spouses and partners in my support group, I've thought a lot about the layers of love and romance. About love and being in love.

A healthy relationship obviously includes both. Your partner is, hopefully, your best friend as well as your lover. We all know that in a long relationship there are days when you can't keep your hands off your partner, when all you want to do is get them alone and make love, and there are days when you can't stand the way they chew their food. But on those days when they are annoying to you, the love is still there. Lust may have taken the day off, but your heart and your soul are still tied to them. It's that love that will endure.

Alzheimer's can destroy many things, but I don't believe it can destroy the deep connection between two souls. It isn't powerful enough to do that. It can and does, however, destroy romance. It's a difficult subject for people to tackle, and there is a great deal of embarrassment around it. It's almost impossible to still be sexually attracted to a partner who is now behaving like a child, who has no capacity to respond in kind. As the disease progresses, they can't bathe themselves or go to the toilet alone. They need to be fed, often by hand because utensils can be dangerous. I'm not sure the shock of this ever wears off, and on the heels of shock often comes depression.

It's a different phase of the relationship, one weighed down by loss. Missing the person you made love with, held through the night, longed for at unexpected hours of the day, is a wound to the heart that can never truly be healed. You watch that person retreat day after day; you slip into bed at night, hoping he or she will already be asleep. Everything is a reminder of what you have lost. The loneliness is vast and unrelenting.

Often, in my support group, the people who were losing a spouse were losing them to early-onset Alzheimer's, which moves at a faster pace. In that situation, trying to process the heartbreak and the loss can feel like a race in which you're always behind. You can only do what you're capable of doing. There will be days when you feel grounded in your love for the person you chose to share your life with, and there will be days when you ache for all that you can no longer share. What I have noticed in people who are faced with this situation is that, over time, they grow more confident in the love that's still there, while at the same time more willing to boldly open the boundaries of their own life. This can mean socializing more without their partner by their side; it can also mean opening themselves to another relationship.

IN 2019, A NEWS STORY came out about B. Smith, the lifestyle guru, and her husband, Dan Gasby.[9] It was already public knowledge that B. had been diagnosed with early-onset Alzheimer's in 2013, when she was sixty-three years old. The couple had been remarkably open and forthright about her disease—how it was affecting their lives, and how they were handling all the changes. They even wrote a book about what they were experiencing in the aftermath of her diagnosis. But this news was different. Gasby revealed that he had fallen in love again, with a woman named Alex Lerner, who stayed often at the house he shared with his wife, and even helped care for her. When I read the story, my first reaction was, "Uh-oh." I knew the floodgates were going to open, with judgment and criticism from all corners, which is exactly what happened. Some of the comments were brutal, both about him and Alex Lerner. I have to assume that most if not all of the people attacking them had no experience with Alzheimer's, because anyone who has been through it knows how complicated life becomes.

To their credit, the couple did not back down. They did interviews, they explained honestly and often eloquently what happens in a relationship when one person is diagnosed with Alzheimer's. What Dan and Alex accomplished was to open a dialogue about the spouses or partners of a person diagnosed with early-onset Alzheimer's and whether or not that partner is entitled to still have joy and companionship in his or her life. In one interview, Dan Gasby spoke about the day he and B. got her diagnosis. He recounted how she said to him that she didn't want him to sacrifice happiness in his own life, that she wanted him to still have a life. He then described the intense loneliness of sitting with her in the evenings when she couldn't have a conversation with him, when she wasn't aware of what was going on in the world or even in the room. For a while, he said, he plunged into depression and tried to self-medicate with alcohol.

He mentioned something that I have said to many caregivers of people with dementia—the statistics of caregivers dying before their loved ones are sobering and alarming. Loneliness and the depression that chases after it can bring on a host of illnesses, and it's not overly dramatic to say that they can kill you. Dan Gasby has said repeatedly that he never stopped loving B.—he cared for her at home with the help of his daughter and subsequently with Alex's help. What he described was a situation that was infused with love from every angle. Was it an unorthodox arrangement? Of course. But there is nothing normal about living with someone who has dementia. The rules that would apply in other circumstances don't fit in the world of dementia.[10]

One of the reasons I wanted to start a support group was that I wanted caregivers to know that they are entitled to still have a fulfilling life. Joy can coexist with grief. Falling in love again doesn't mean you no longer love the person who is ill. Loneliness doesn't have to be your prison and your punishment. When missing the person who is ill becomes overwhelming, isn't it better to be able to fall into the arms of someone who loves you and cares about you, someone who understands? The alternative is to be eroded by sorrow and emptied out by loss. It's too easy to slip into that reality and end up wrapped in despair, unable to move. It's hard work to reach for happiness when sorrow is pulling at you from every corner, harder still to open your heart to new love when you're aching for the person you still love but whom you barely recognize. I don't believe we were put on this earth to surrender to pain—acknowledge it, yes, and learn from it, absolutely. We are meant instead to find our way through it to an open field where other possibilities await us.

B. Smith died in February 2020. She was seventy years old. People will remember her work as a lifestyle guru, but a huge part of her legacy will be how she and her husband took hold of the disease that claimed her at a young age and turned her experience into a life lesson for others. Even in the vast, empty spaces of Alzheimer's she was still smiling. She and her husband still found joy in life. They proved that Alzheimer's couldn't kill that.

"He who learns must suffer. And even in our sleep pain that cannot forget falls drop by drop upon the heart, and in our own despair, against our will, comes wisdom to us by the awful grace of God."   —AESCHYLUS

WHEN THINGS GET
OUT OF CONTROL

CHAPTER 11

Calling Adult Protective Services

One of the stark realities of dementia is that sometimes things go horribly wrong, despite the best intentions of caring family members. This can happen at any time, even in the early stages, but generally more problems erupt as the disease progresses. There are several scenarios in which reporting to Adult Protective Services might be warranted.[1] The person with dementia might already be involved in an inappropriate romantic relationship, or someone new might come into their life after they have been diagnosed—someone who is conniving and intends to take advantage of them. Dementia doesn't allow them to see what's obvious to everyone else. There are also situations in which a family member is neglectful or even abusive. According to a person I know who contacted Adult Protective Services, he was told by the responding APS worker that the majority of calls to the agency have to do with neglect by a caregiver.

Sometimes the problem doesn't involve a second party. Rather, the individual who has been diagnosed becomes a danger to him- or herself by refusing care, rejecting the idea of moving to an assisted care facility or even to the home of a relative. To an Alzheimer's patient, home may become a fortress, but it can also be extremely dangerous if that person lives there alone.

Every state has a version of APS, and there are some differences state to state, but the basics are the same. If a report is made that a person over the age of sixty is being mistreated or neglected, if there is suspicion of abuse—physical, financial, or emotional—APS will open an investigation. If they decide that the report warrants it, they will follow up and conduct an interview with the person who is reportedly being abused and also with appropriate family members and caregivers. In severe cases, APS has the option of involving the police. The same sequence happens if the person refuses to leave home. APS will investigate whether that individual is a danger to him- or herself.[2]

In the realm of dementia, things can get tricky. For example: a woman's divorced mother, who has been diagnosed with Alzheimer's, has been seeing a man who her daughter believes is exploiting her financially and is not properly caring for her. He goes to doctors' appointments with her, has put himself in charge of her medications, and makes unilateral decisions about what she should or shouldn't take. Her mother is basically supporting him, yet even if there is financial proof that money has been taken by this man, her mother claims she wanted to give it to him and doesn't see that he is neglecting her needs. She might be in denial about the severity of her dementia and might feel that she doesn't need anyone's help, another huge obstacle.

The daughter can file a report with APS, and probably should. If APS feels that there is enough there to investigate, they will make an appointment to speak to the mother. But if she tells them that everything is fine, that she isn't being financially abused, that there is no neglect, the person from APS has to accept that. Of course, APS also has to consider the daughter's complaint. But they can't order the man out of her mother's life. And if he is guilty of financial abuse, he is probably good at conning people and making himself look innocent. A situation like this can get very complicated and the results are not always what the complainant wants. But filing a claim at least establishes a record if things continue to get worse.

Other precautions can be taken. Family members can speak to the bank to make them aware of their concerns and suspicions regarding their loved one, so the bank can be on alert. There are also elder-care attorneys who specialize in these complex situations.

On occasion, someone may wish to file a complaint with APS anonymously, which can be done. For example, if a family member is being neglectful or abusive, other relatives might want to get help from APS but have their identity remain confidential to avoid an explosive situation. Or a neighbor might see things that are concerning but might not want to get personally involved. APS will investigate anonymous complaints.

Sadly, there are too many cases in which someone with dementia is put under the care of a family member, might even be living in that family member's home, and is found wandering around the neighborhood, or they appear unwashed and unkempt. That is absolutely cause for reporting to APS, and anyone can do it—a neighbor, even a delivery person or the mail carrier. However, if APS comes and is not allowed into the home, they can't force their way in. Legally, if they feel it's necessary, they will then have to involve the police and get a warrant.

Once inside the home, APS inspects the environment and assesses the condition, physical and mental, of the dementia patient. They take photographs inside the home to document if it's safe for that individual to live there. They try to determine if the individual is competent to keep him- or herself clean, knows how to use the kitchen appliances, understands what to eat and what not to put in their mouth. They will look for signs of abuse or neglect. If there is a family member with power of attorney, they will almost certainly want to speak with that person.

When APS determines that the individual with dementia needs to be in a facility, and family members, even with power of attorney, have been neglectful, a guardian must be appointed. This requires going to court. Elder-care attorneys handle this. The patient must be deemed by a court to be incapable of caring for themselves, and the guardian does not necessarily have to be a family member. It might be a social worker or someone else appointed by the court.[3]

A situation I heard about often in the support group, which I think happens frequently, is that someone diagnosed with Alzheimer's or some other form of dementia refuses to leave home and refuses to allow a caregiver to come in. I have heard of occasions when APS arrived to speak with the person and were not allowed through the front door. I have also heard of dementia patients lying, claiming that they were being abused by a family member when that was untrue. Sometimes the accused family member wasn't able to get inside the house either. APS agents are trained to assess situations in which someone with dementia is making claims—that they are fine, or that they are being abused. But no system is perfect, and the agents aren't psychic, so this can be an extremely stressful experience. A lot can go wrong.

The circumstances that make it advisable to call APS or retain an elder-care attorney can push family members to the breaking point. It takes an already tense, emotional situation and ramps it up. However, the cost of not taking action can be severe.

Someone in my support group, whose parent was refusing both to leave home and to allow anyone in, practically cried out in exasperation, "Why can't I get through to my parent?"—beating themselves up for not being able to solve this crisis. I knew that the relationship between the two of them had never been a close and communicative one. I was reminded of something Marianne Williamson said in a lecture many years ago. She was talking about the work she did with AIDS patients at the beginning of her career and she said that once, in prayer, she asked God why she couldn't just touch someone with AIDS and cure them. She was, after all, lecturing about miracles; she knew that miraculous healings had happened throughout history, and she believed in them, so why couldn't she produce one? What she heard back, in her mind, was, "Why can't you be calm when your mother calls?"

We often think that we should be able to do some monumental thing when we haven't even mastered small steps, like staying calm when our mother calls. This is when a logical, albeit unpleasant, solution like calling APS is the best course of action. Sometimes you simply can't fix things on your own.

⁊⊘

REMEMBER THAT APS IS a government agency, so they are not always going to be as quick or thorough as you would like. If you have to go this route, you have to be proactive and patient. You may need to make a number of phone calls before you get a response. But as I said before, there is little choice if your loved one is being abused in some way or is refusing care in his or her home.

It may seem impossible to find gratitude in these circumstances but consider: What if there were no agency to call? What if you were left on your own while your elderly parent was locked inside the home, refusing care? Or was being financially or physically abused by another family member, a hired caregiver, or someone else who was let into their life?

In situations of abuse, always contact APS and file a report. If you are certain that physical abuse or neglect is taking place, you might want to insist that the police be involved. In the event of a loved one shunning care at home and refusing to leave and go to a safer place, try all other remedies first—family intervention, the intervention of a priest, minister, or rabbi if that is appropriate. If none of those work, then a decision to involve APS is the best you can do. The possible tragic scenarios of leaving a dementia patient alone are numerous and frightening, and you would never want any of them on your conscience.

Sometimes people have promised their parents that they will always be able to stay at home, no matter what. You can't undo what has already been said, but if you are thinking of making such a promise, it's better not to. You have no idea what turns life may take. And while it sounds noble and generous to assure your parents that they will never have to leave their home, it might not turn out to be realistic. I know people who made that pledge and then had to confront the reality that Alzheimer's made it impossible for their parent to remain at home and the only responsible choice was to move them to a facility where they would get constant care. They could only hope that their promise would be forgotten.

Unfortunately, someone with dementia often doesn't forget what you wish they would forget.

"Find the place inside where there is joy, and the joy will burn out the pain."   —JOSEPH CAMPBELL

CHAPTER 12

They Were So Much Better Yesterday

A man whose mother has been diagnosed with Alzheimer's feels that they have at least settled into a dependable rhythm. She has remained relatively stable for nearly a year. When she made it clear she did not want to leave her home, he hired a part-time caregiver to keep her company for four hours a day. He arranged to have prepared food available so that all she has to do is put it in the microwave. Usually, when the caregiver leaves in the afternoon, his mother is ready to take a nap. He checks on her when he gets back from work, sits with her for a while, and leaves her watching television. She forgets names and dates and gets confused sometimes, but seems to have adapted to the pattern they have established.

Then one day he arrives at her house after work, as he always does, and finds the front door wide open. She's gone. He calls the caregiver and is told that his mother was fine when she finished her shift. Nothing seemed different. He knocks on neighbors' doors, but they didn't see her. He calls the police and reports her missing; he has to tell them that she has Alzheimer's. Hours pass and he doesn't want to go home in case she returns.

Long after the sun has set, a car pulls up and his mother gets out. A man has driven her home. He found her in the parking lot of a grocery store, looking lost and confused. She didn't remember her address, the man says, but she had her purse with her and she still had an old driver's license. Now she seems unfazed, completely unaware of what has happened. The man thanks the stranger, but a nagging thought makes him wonder if she had cash in her wallet and if it's still there. There is no way to know because she has no idea what was in her wallet.

He insists that she come home with him and spend the night there, giving her no room to refuse. But now what? He has to work, he can't get a full-time caregiver by the next day. Suddenly, everything that was orderly in his world is in shambles. He will have to beg for some time off from work to hire more care; he is realizing that he can't be sure his mother will sleep through the night and not get up and walk out of the house.

He is weighed down, not only by the circumstances, but by a feeling of failure—a feeling that he should have known this was coming, should have prepared for it. The reality that his mother might not be able to stay in her home is descending on him. The only way he will be able to afford a facility for her is by selling her house, and how will he explain that to her?

This is just one example of the quick turns that Alzheimer's, or any kind of dementia, can take. It's human nature to slip into a routine, to feel on some level that life will coast along in a familiar way. We tend to believe there will be signs that something is about to change. Perhaps, we think, our loved one will suddenly have a larger-than-usual memory lapse, signaling that the disease is worsening. That might happen, but it also might not. Alzheimer's forges ahead with no predictability and no signposts along the way. The victim can go from someone who is still capable of fixing their own meals to someone who walks out of the house, believing that they are heading back to their childhood home.

Even though it feels unnatural, and we resist it, preparing for what is inevitable is the best way to avoid a panic situation. When disasters, either real, imagined, or likely, are crowding in on you, it's hard to think straight. It's easier to set things in motion for the next phase when you're in a calmer frame of mind. If you know that down the line, the only way to afford a facility for your parent is to sell their home, line up a realtor ahead of time, study the market, and prepare. Check out care facilities, find out which ones you don't care for and which might be good for your parent. You don't have to tell your parent—in fact, I suggest that you don't—but having the groundwork done will ready you for what is coming.

Look clearly at all the things that can possibly happen—all the dangers that a person with dementia can stumble into. I have heard of someone with Alzheimer's cranking up the microwave to a dangerous setting and then forgetting about it, fortunately blowing out the circuit before the house caught fire. I know of a woman who drank shampoo because the bottle looked similar to the Evian water bottle she usually drank from, a man who walked out of the house and tried to cross the freeway, and a woman who got lost a block from her house and accepted a ride from a stranger who later returned, seeing her as an easy mark.

Of course, even if you anticipate every possible catastrophe you can think of, things can still happen. You simply cannot anticipate what dementia is going to do or when it's going to do it. It's a strange balance, learning to live in the present moment—which is where the person with Alzheimer's usually lives—and planning for a future that can look like a tangled mess. You will be blindsided at times, that's a given. Plan as much as you can, think ahead as much as you can, and then just remember to breathe.

✧

WITH MY FATHER, as I've said before, we had a built-in guard rail with the Secret Service on the premises. He wasn't going to wander off, but that didn't mean he couldn't get into trouble. There came a point when—as happens with most people who have Alzheimer's—he had difficulty recognizing certain objects. He would stare at them, making it obvious that he wasn't sure what a fork was, or a comb. It's very common for people with Alzheimer's to start putting things in their mouth, just as young children do, so that's a risk that needs to be anticipated.

Another indication that my father had fallen off the plateau he had remained on for several years was that his cognition didn't just splinter at the end of day. Sundowning may become more of an all-day event as the disease worsens. Those who experience it are still usually best in the morning, but the rest of the day is up and down. You can no longer depend on time of day as a way to gauge how your loved one is going to act.

My father's pattern of going into the office for a few hours every weekday continued for several years. Visitors were carefully screened and allowed to spend a few minutes with him, have their pictures taken, and interact with him. There was little else for him to do there. One of the saddest things about visiting him in the office was seeing his desk. It had nothing on it except a pen holder, a clock, and a yellow pad on which he sketched. Amazingly, he still remembered how to compose the doodles he had always drawn—figures, faces, sometimes horses, always done quickly as if he had been a cartoonist in a past life. But the emptiness of the space in front of him as he sat at his desk hurt my heart every time.

In letting him still go to the office, my mother was walking a fine line between giving him some kind of normalcy—a piece of the life he had known—and protecting his dignity. I am almost certain that it was one particular office visit that made her decide it was time to keep him home. In 1998, when the aircraft carrier the USS *Ronald Reagan* was nearly completed, several military men made an appointment to see my father and show him a model—sort of a mini unveiling. They put the model on a table, removed the covering they had over it, and told him what it was and what it would be called. My father looked at it and asked, "Can you ride horses on it?" No one ever told me if anyone responded to him, although I have to assume that someone said something. I laughed when I heard the story because it was sweet and endearing, and actually could have been a joke that my father might have made in healthier times. My mother, however, was not amused. She found it embarrassing, and it seemed to catapult her into deciding that he should no longer go into the office.

This was another instance when I felt acutely the sadness of my family—that we never discussed decisions as a group. The rest of us were either informed, or not informed, about decisions my mother made, and she never seemed to realize that her journey didn't have to be so lonely. I believe all of us would have rallied around her, despite our fractured past, but it wasn't to be. My mother would end up dying alone in the middle of the night, never knowing that she had great-grandchildren. Michael's son, Cameron, had married and had two little girls, but my mother had banished Michael and his family. She never visited Seattle, where Ron had lived for decades, so she had no idea what his life was like there. I've sometimes wondered if we compose the ending of our life with every choice we make.

Once my father's daily routine changed to really no routine at all, the male caregiver who had been hired for about four hours a day was replaced by a woman who had nursed my father back to health after he was shot in 1981. She was still a registered nurse but no longer working at a hospital, so she was free to come live at my parents' house and care for him. She sat beside my father at the dinner table, and it was another sad milestone when I dined with them one night and watched her cut up his food for him.

Soon he grew silent, talking very little, and his eyes revealed that he was far away. Wherever he had drifted off to seemed to be a peaceful place. If there was any consolation for the worsening of the disease, it was that he no longer had spells of looking frightened or confused. He had been carried out to deeper waters far past those emotions.

One night when I went to my parents' house for dinner, a supermoon was rising in the sky. As we sat at the table, it shone through the plate-glass windows, taking over a large area of the sky. A supermoon coincides with perigee, when the moon moves closest to the earth in its elliptical orbit. My father would have loved talking about it in another time. Thinking I might slip past the disease for a moment, I said, "Dad, look at the moon. It's a supermoon. It's closer to the earth right now."

He glanced up but I'm not sure his eyes focused, and he didn't say anything; he just paused for a second and looked back down at his plate. When I was a little girl, I thought my father hung the moon. Now, I couldn't share the majesty of it with him.

THE REALIZATION THAT THE disease is getting worse, however it happens, is one of the hardest junctures for family and loved ones. No matter how clear-headed we have been, how realistic our inner dialogue—telling ourselves that of course the disease will progress—we tend to latch on to where the person is in the early stages. It's almost a survival instinct. Our brains know things will get worse, but our emotions don't listen.

With the exception of early-onset Alzheimer's and frontotemporal dementia, people with dementia commonly do remain on a plateau for a while after the disease is diagnosed. So it's natural for caregivers to become used to it, almost lulled by it, to think, "If they just stay here, like this, I can handle it." It's also common, if the person is elderly, to have a slightly uncomfortable thought that you tend to keep to yourself: because of their age, death is imminent. Maybe death will come before the disease gets worse, sparing them the late stages.

My father was eighty-three when he was diagnosed, and I definitely had that thought. I wanted him to be spared the advanced progress of the disease. Death seemed the kinder alternative. Some people in my support group reluctantly admitted that they, too, thought about this. It's a very difficult thing to admit, even to oneself. We have complicated and conflicting ideas about death, and most of us are self-conscious about it. So, to say, "Yes, I see death as a reprieve from the worst stages of this disease" makes us either feel guilty or at least wonder if we should feel guilty. The truth is, we would all be more at peace if we were more comfortable talking about death—about our fears, our imaginings, the questions that haunt us, and even the idea that it can sometimes be a blessing. But our culture, more than some others, has made death an almost forbidden subject.

Then dementia enters our life, and death becomes a thought we harbor in the deepest chambers of our hearts—maybe my loved one will leave before being taken away from all he or she has known. And because we have this thought, it hits us hard when the person falls from a months- or even year-long plateau and gets conspicuously worse. Our fears charge in, our hope diminishes, and we feel more acutely the emptiness of who our loved one once was. It's the stage at which the full reality of the disease crashes down on us.

※

As I write this, the world is in the midst of the global coronavirus pandemic. Entire states are effectively shut down. In California, where I live, grocery store shelves are empty. Stores are closed. People are frightened. You can feel the fear and anxiety everywhere, as well as the sense of helplessness. There is nowhere we can go to escape this virus, no other state or country—it has made its way around the globe. The absence of life as we knew it yawns around us, reminds us every hour of what we no longer have right now. Every morning I wake up and remember that this is really happening. The days are quiet; even the skies have been silenced since most planes are grounded. I remember the long-ago mornings when I woke and brushed up against the knowledge that my father, the elusive man I had always longed to know better, was being stolen away, and there was nothing I could do to change that.

When coronavirus first hit, I thought about how the cocktail of feelings—fear, anxiety, sorrow—live in a familiar place inside all of us who have experienced the challenge of an incurable illness. Dementia ushers in a pervasive sense of helplessness. It's there at the start, when the diagnosis is handed down, and it's there during the early stages. But at the moment you realize the disease is accelerating and you have no idea what's going to happen next, it envelops you.

There is one marked difference between the helplessness of having a loved one with dementia and the helplessness that abounds in the Covid pandemic—in the latter, everyone is affected. When we pass people outside on walks, moving over to keep a safe distance from one another, there is still some emotional connection, an acknowledgment that we are all feeling the same anxiety and stress. Everyone on earth is going through this to one degree or another. Strangers lock eyes, exchange greetings; before they would have just passed by. We say, "How are you?" to people we don't know and we really do want to hear the answer. In contrast, having a loved one with Alzheimer's, while not unique, feels isolating, as if no one else can relate to our experience.

A couple whom I met when they came to my support group in its early years and who kept coming religiously every week, have allowed me to share their story, a powerful illustration of the learning curve that Alzheimer's asks you to undergo, as well as the stages of grief and loss.

Shortly after they married, the couple I'll call Cara and Thomas moved Cara's mother, Michelle, into their home. They had two children, a boy and a girl, and Michelle was an attentive grandmother. Cara and Thomas run their own business, so having her there made their lives easier. The first night they came to the support group, they described some of the changes they were seeing in Michelle. I asked them where she was right then, while they were at the group. They said the kids were now older and already out of the house, so she was at home, by herself. Cara added that she was fine. My cofacilitator and I said in unison, "No, she's not."

Here is how Cara describes the trajectory of the illness:

My mother had lived with us for thirty years, freed up our lives so we could work, and so that we could take the occasional trip, just the two of us. That balance that Mom brought to the house was one of the beautiful things we always talked to people about. We called it the joy of a three-generation household. Yes, we related to the term "sandwich generation," where we were taking care of both a younger and an older generation, but we felt we were living the best life. It was such a pleasure to have her stories of "the old days," and the kids loved the way she joked around and protected them (from us, the mean ogre parents who had— God forbid—rules!) when they did something wrong. However, as time went on, having my mother was in many ways like having a third, but grown, child.

We started noticing that things were getting odd. She scraped all the paint off the hood of our car with a credit card, thinking she was cleaning up after an egg was thrown at it by kids on Halloween night. We had a dark green car when we left for work one day, and we came home to a black car—the undercoat. When we asked what happened, she didn't have a clue. And then there was the time she scraped all the lacquer off our kitchen cabinets, thinking she was cleaning them. We didn't know it at the time, but that ultra-obsessive behavior is typical of dementia patients. We took her in for an evaluation after these incidents and were told that she had Mild Cognitive Impairment and that we should watch her closely.

Then she had some illnesses that required surgery. That's when her health went downhill fast. We didn't know at the time that anesthesia significantly worsens dementia symptoms. Suddenly, she was moody, had trouble sleeping, was easily frustrated. But she was still driving. We were in denial about how bad things were. She seemed competent in so many ways, but actually she wasn't at all. Our daughter, who had gone to college, came home and observed that things with Mom had changed drastically. Then another friend, who hadn't seen Mom in a year, visited and said the same thing. That's when we knew we had to take the car keys away. She rebelled, got angry—her freedom was gone. But then she calmed down. It was hard but we did it. One stress was lifted.

When we had twenty-four-hour caregivers in the house, everyone was miserable. We couldn't find the right person. We tried a live-in for salary plus room and board, but that was a drag. Mom hated all of the caregivers. Again, her freedom, her privacy, her world all suffered. Moving her into a care facility was the best solution, but that was fraught at first too.

Finally, we found the right place. They agreed to paint the room the same color as her room at home; we moved in all her furniture (that was like a scene from Keystone Cops) in one day. I took her shopping while Thomas and our friends moved her furniture and décor to the new place. Then I took her to lunch and gave her a relaxant that her doctor had prescribed, took her to the home, and left her there. She thought she was home. It was great, or so we thought. We were advised to not see her for two

weeks so she could adjust; during those two weeks she would call
us crying, screaming, frantic. But then she eased into the place.
We finally visited. She was still angry, but we got through it. She
came to love the facility and the caregivers, and she still loved us.
(It took me three years in the support group to get over the guilt.)

I remember well Cara's persistent guilt. But I also remember
how diligently she worked on dismantling it. She knew, intellectually, that placing her mother in a facility where she would get round-
the-clock care was the best choice. There was no way Michelle could
have stayed in their home without catastrophic consequences. But
our emotions always trail behind what we know to be true.

Michelle lived out the rest of her days in the care facility with
her family visiting often and the familiar objects of a lifetime around
her. It had been a long process of admitting that things had deteri-
orated to accepting that the best choice for all of them was a care
facility. Interestingly, Cara and Thomas initially came to the support
group after seeing an ad in the UCLA paper. Cara said, "I thought
maybe it would make me feel better." Neither of them anticipated
going on a long journey of discovery and companionship, a journey
that would shift their thinking, challenge them, and ultimately calm
their hearts.

※

IN JANUARY 2001 my father fell at my parents' home and broke
his hip. He hadn't been going into the office for several years; in fact,
he didn't really have any kind of schedule. He would often sleep late
into the morning. He was still taken on walks in the afternoon and
he now had rotating shifts of caregivers during the day, so that there
was always someone watching him. They put a pressure mat at his

bedside: it emitted a sound if he got out of bed and stepped onto the mat. But for some reason, on one particular morning, someone forgot to turn it on. Late in the morning one of the caregivers peeked into the bedroom to see if he was awake and found him lying on the floor beside the bed. He wasn't making a sound, though he must have been in pain. An ambulance took him to Saint John's Hospital, where they discovered that his hip was badly broken and he would need an operation. I got a call from a woman who works for my parents, as did other family members, and in an odd dance that we'd all become familiar with, we got updates on our father's condition by watching the news. On the second day we were allowed to see him.

Saint John's had become somewhat familiar to me at that time; my sister Maureen was there being treated for the melanoma that had returned with a vengeance. The cancer had spread throughout her body, but she was emphatic that she didn't want to give in, so they were trying all sorts of medications including thalidomide, which they thought—experimentally—might eradicate some of the tumors. She was a few floors away from my father, but because she was hooked up to so many machines, she wasn't able to see him. It was heartbreaking to witness her grief, her anger, her desperation. I thought then, and still think, that she was holding fast to life because she didn't want to die before our father. Her situation was basically hopeless, and I wished in my heart that she would accept that reality and soften her resistance to death. I wanted an easier ending for her. I wanted her to "go gentle into that good night," as Dylan Thomas put it. But it wasn't to be. She would get to see my father one last time at my parents' house, after he got home from the hospital and she was released to go home to Sacramento, where she would die seven months later, in August.

Going into my father's hospital room the day after his surgery is an image that has stayed with me. I noticed his paleness, which was to be expected, and his frailty. In the harsh fluorescent light his skin almost looked translucent. But what registered most forcefully was the fact that his eyes looked even more distant. I stroked his hand and it felt cold. I reached for his eyes with mine, but he was light-years away. I thought they must have medicated him for pain—that could account for how different he looked. Also, the shock, the dis-orientation, of falling and ending up in the hospital could certainly have been factors.

It was not the first time I had walked into a hospital room to see my father. Twenty years earlier, in 1981, after John Hinckley shot him, I approached his hospital bed and searched his eyes. That day, I saw a light in them, different from anything I had seen before. It seemed almost other-worldly. I have believed since that day that my father had a near-death experience. It may not have been docu-mented, he may not have clinically flatlined, but, to me, his eyes told the story. In the days after, he recounted waking up in the Intensive Care Unit, seeing men in white standing around his bed, and asking them if he was alive. The strange thing about that story is, doctors wear scrubs, not white jackets, in the ICU. It was further evidence to me that what I had seen in his eyes was the look of a man who had crossed over and returned.

When I saw my father in the hospital after he had his hip repaired, the look in his eyes was different. There was something per-manent and vast about the distance. I felt as if he wasn't coming back to where he was before he fell. I learned years later, in some of the research I did for Beyond Alzheimer's, and also by talking to cofa-cilitators in the medical field, that anesthesia quite often worsens the symptoms of dementia.[4] This does not mean that anesthesia causes dementia—there is no evidence to suggest that it does. But someone who already has dementia and is put under general anesthesia may not emerge from it at the same cognitive level as before the surgery. The same holds true for head injuries. If the injury is severe enough, the symptoms of a dementia patient who falls and hits his head will very probably worsen.

My father definitely changed after his surgery. It was noticeable to all of us, but I think we assumed it was caused by the trauma of what he'd gone through. Even if we had known about the link between anesthesia and symptoms of dementia, there was nothing we could have done differently. His hip was badly broken and needed to be repaired surgically; there was simply no choice but to put him under general anesthesia.

What dominated everyone's attention at that point was his physical state and the changes that needed to be made in his home environment. He got a walker and was going to need physical therapy at home. He would need round-the-clock nursing care. At some point, the decision was made to put him in a hospital bed in the room that was once his study, but would now, and for the remainder of his days, just be called "his room."

He was at this stage when I had my biggest challenge in keeping hold of the faith I had depended upon, the faith that told me I could reach past Alzheimer's and somehow find my father. In the decade of his illness, this period was my dark night of the soul. Tears came, predictably, at night, and were often followed by nightmares. In one dream, we were back at the Pacific Palisades house I grew up in. My parents and my brother Ron were there, along with one of our dogs who, when she grew old, was in so much pain that we had to make the difficult decision to put her down. In my dream, I thought we were taking her to the vet for that purpose, but my father said no, you're taking me to be put down. I woke up breathless and crying, afraid to go back to sleep because the dream was so real.

I wished so much that I could share what I saw as a spiritual crisis with someone from my family, but that was impossible. My brother Ron is an atheist. If I reached out to Michael, my mother would ostracize me. Maureen was dying. And discussing spiritual matters with my mother was something I couldn't even conceive of. I had, years earlier, decided to not burden friends with my journey through the world of Alzheimer's, so I was very much alone. The only person to whom I had ever brought spiritual questions and dilemmas was my father.

Even as a little girl, I questioned him often about God. There was a hill behind our house where he used to take me to fly kites. On one of those days—a windy blue afternoon—I lifted myself up on my tiptoes, reached my arms up to the sky, and asked him how high I'd have to reach up to touch God. He knelt down beside me and explained that I didn't need to reach up at all. God is everywhere, he said. Everywhere in the world and everywhere inside you, you just need to talk to him. It's one of those memories that's carved into me—my father kneeling on the dirt path, white muscular clouds floating above us—and a lesson about God that I would remember all my life.

But, so many years later, at the stage of my father's disease when he had drifted light-years away, God felt far away to me as well. I decided the only thing I could do was try to resurrect the faith that had grounded me up to that point, and I needed to go to my father for help. On the days I visited my parents, I would choose times when my mother was busy and then ask the nurses if I could have some private time with my father. Once we were alone, I spoke to him in whispers. I told him many things—how I was sorry for the ways in which I had hurt him with my rebelliousness, how my heart held fast to the lessons he had taught me as a child, lessons about faith and trust in a God who sees everything. I told him I felt lost right then, as if faith had abandoned me, and I wished I could have a sign in my life as he did when he was a young man and he woke up feeling invisible hands on his shoulders. I loved that story, I made him tell it to me often. He would describe how he sat up in bed, feeling enveloped by the most profound sense of love and protection, and he knew it was God's hands he was feeling on his shoulders. All my life I've wished for a sign. As I told him about that, something glimmered in his eyes, and I heard deep inside myself a message that said signs were everywhere—I just had to pay attention.

I realized that faith isn't an easy thing to keep alive and hold onto. It can slip away from us, and then we have to claw our way back to it, often over the treacherous terrain of our own doubts. But maybe I hadn't lost as much as I thought I had. It was faith that took me to my father's bedside, looking for him to remind me again that God is everywhere. I don't need to stand on my tiptoes, I don't need to reach up my arms, I just need to trust. I've never had the dramatic experience my father had waking up to the feeling of ethereal hands on his shoulders. I've had to look harder, wrestle with doubts. Sometimes faith is only a tiny flame resisting the wind. And sometimes God is there in the faint glimmer passing across blue eyes that have faded and turned inward.

I think of those times in my father's room, sometimes sitting in complete silence, as the deepest and most honest conversations we ever had. They grounded me for what was to come, and I never again doubted that his soul rested calm and healthy beyond the fog of Alzheimer's. It is not lost on me that this man who I spent my life wanting to be closer to, to know better, took up residence in the part of my spirit that needed him the most. He brought me back to God when I felt abandoned, just as he had piloted my way to God when I was a child. After so many decades of feeling that I couldn't find my father, I realized he was there all along, just not in the ways I had yearned for. He was not the accessible father, participating in his children's lives, going to athletic events and school performances. He didn't know the names of my friends or what my interests were. But he was a voice inside me when I was a teenager strung out on drugs, a lost kid who couldn't figure out why she should live. My father was a thousand miles away, in another state that night, having no idea what I was going through, but his voice was lodged in my heart and it pulled me back from the edge. He was there when I asked for God's forgiveness for all the ways I had hurt him publicly with my ill-thought-out political protests. He had told me as a child that God forgives all His children who ask for forgiveness, and in a place far beyond my tears, I heard his echo. Even when Alzheimer's silenced his voice, I heard him.

Our parents don't always show up for us in the ways that we want them to. But sometimes, if we're lucky and if we pay close attention, we can find them in hidden pockets of our lives where they were waiting all along. Some of us are left with just the memory of isolated moments with a parent who we could never get close to, but those moments matter. If you search through your history with that parent, odds are you will find at least one time when he or she turned to you with tenderness and love. Even if it was only once, it's a memory you need to shine light on and look at often. I am fortunate in having many memories of my father that still give me sustenance—maybe not as many as some people have with a parent, but enough. It was a different story with my mother, and at the end of her life, when I composed my eulogy for her, I admit that I struggled to unearth moments of tenderness. But there were some, and I still think of them. One benefit of doing this is that you get to see what your parent missed out on. There was love between you; they just chose not to nurture it. Now, as they are leaving this world on the tide of a disease that will never allow them to grow and change, you have a chance to feel compassion and sympathy for them.

People who are losing a parent to dementia usually get to this point when the disease worsens, when past and present collide and the history they have shared is like a tableau in front of them. It's both a painful and a pivotal time. How you choose to respond to it will determine how you go through the rest of the journey.

❦

AFTER MY FATHER'S SURGERY, a valiant effort was made to have him do physical therapy so he would be able to walk again, maybe even go for walks around the local park, which had become a dependable outing for him. I don't remember now how it started to become clear that this was not going to work. He was tired, he didn't want to do physical therapy. He wanted to sleep and stare into the distance as the sun moved across the sky. He was ninety, and he had an incurable illness that was claiming more of him with each passing season. Our desire was not shared by him and, to my mother's credit, she realized that.

Often we have an agenda for our loved one that has more to

do with us than it does with them. If my father could walk again, if he could return to what he did before he fell and had surgery on his hip, then it would seem as if we had gotten some power over Alzheimer's—as if we had won a round in the boxing match that we would ultimately lose. But you don't get power over Alzheimer's. As I've said, the disease is running the show.

Over the years I have listened to people talk about how they think it would be good for their loved one to keep going for walks or keep dressing themselves when there is evidence that they no longer know how. Sometimes people have encouraged a parent or spouse to reactivate an interest in gardening, certain that they are operating on a basis of what's best for their loved one. But when it's gently pointed out to them that maybe they're trying to assuage their own fears, their own despair, a light goes on. Usually, anyway; some people get mad at me.

If your loved one is elderly and ill and doesn't want to walk and exercise their muscles, let them be. I believe strongly that somewhere in their soul they are preparing for the end they know is coming. If they want to sit by the window and stare outside, what's the harm? They don't have to have a schedule anymore; they don't have to put in a certain number of steps on their Fitbit. They're facing the end of their life, and the rest of us need to honor that.

Years ago, I knew a woman who was dying of lung cancer. There was nothing else the doctors could do. I was having dinner with her and another friend, when she lit a cigarette. The friend was shocked and expressed his surprise. The woman smiled as she exhaled smoke and said, "What does it matter? I'm dying. This makes me happy." She had the ability to tell us how she was feeling, whereas people with Alzheimer's cannot, but that doesn't mean that they aren't reflecting on death deep inside and leaning into what makes them happy. They might cherish the solitude of simply sitting by a window for hours.

So, if my father made it obvious that he was unhappy doing physical therapy, the nurses were told to back off. This started to happen every time. As it progressed, he became essentially bedridden. He couldn't use the walker and there seemed no point in putting him in a wheelchair since moving him from the bed to the wheelchair was difficult and uncomfortable for him. Around this same time, my mother revealed that she had been told to expect that he would only live another three months. That's the conventional wisdom when an elderly person with serious health issues breaks a hip; that's the time frame doctors are familiar with. My father lived three more years, but those years were spent in a hospital bed in front of a bank of windows that looked out on oak trees and a changing sky. He watched seasons pass, he watched storms rumble across the sky and sunlight slant its way through tree branches. And he said very little. There was a portrait of my mother in his room, which he sometimes stared at, and often when I came over for dinner we would eat on fold-up tables in his room.

When Maureen died, I asked my mother if she had told my father about her passing. She said no, because he wouldn't understand. I waited until I had another private visit with him, and I whispered to him that Maureen had gone home to God—that's how my father described death to me when I was a child. He looked at me, blinked his eyes a couple of times, but I saw no glimmer of recognition, no sign that I had gotten beyond the veil of Alzheimer's. It didn't matter, though—my faith had been restored and I believed that he did hear me. I told him that he and Maureen would see each other again on the other side, that she'd probably be waiting for him and would have many things to tell him, which she always seemed to when she was alive. I had no plans to ever bring up the subject again, and I never did. But I felt strongly that he deserved to know that his daughter had died. I didn't want to step into the quicksand of "He won't understand."

Years later, when people in my support group were in a similar situation and wondered if they should tell their loved one that a family member or friend had died, I always stressed that it depended on where their loved one was in the disease. If there was a chance that they would keep asking about that person, then it was risky. If there was a chance they would perseverate on it, and not be able to move past the fact that someone close to them had died, it might be best to not tell them. In my father's case, he had drifted so far away that those scenarios were unlikely. I felt that on the level at which I believed he could hear me, it was right to tell him, but only that one time. Like many other aspects of Alzheimer's, it's a judgment call. You need to determine what's going to be best, and the least stressful, both for your loved one and for you.

"There is no teacher more discriminating or transforming than loss."
                                                              —Pat Conroy

CHAPTER 13

The Battle Over Bathing
(and Other Health Dilemmas)

With all the uncertainties and surprises that Alzheimer's brings in the realm of behavior, there is one thing you can count on—at a certain point, your loved one will rebel at the idea of going into the shower. It won't happen early on in the disease, but eventually it will. I think we avoided reaching that point with my father because of his fall, which resulted in him becoming bedridden. Prior to that, a chair had been put into the shower for his safety, since he had lost strength and balance. He still willingly went in at bath time, but I'm fairly certain that would have changed if he hadn't fallen and broken his hip, because this behavior is so common.

Why? There is no concrete reason that anyone can point to. Maybe water itself becomes frightening, or the enclosure of a shower. No one knows. I've heard story after story from caregivers whose loved one suddenly reacted in fear when it came time to step into the shower, although days earlier they were fine with it. I tend to think that the water coming down on them becomes frightening. And the fear can be explosive. One man told me about his eighty-six-year-old arthritic mother who had Alzheimer's and refused to get into the shower; she hit her caregiver in the face and broke the woman's nose; the caregiver quit after that.

Elderly dementia patients who don't seem to have the strength for a full-blown tantrum can erupt violently. Many people say that they aren't worried about their mother or father hurting themselves or someone else if they become enraged because their parents are in their eighties or nineties and have little physical strength, so "what damage can they do?" The answer is a lot. It doesn't matter how old or infirm a person is: in an adrenalized state they can still do things that ordinarily they would be incapable of. I'm not sure that your eighty-year-old mother who has Alzheimer's could lift up a car, but I am sure that she could smash a lamp on your head if enough adrenaline were released in her body. Generally speaking, the fear over getting into the shower tends to be extreme. And once it's there, it doesn't go away.

So, what to do? What you shouldn't do is waste time trying to talk the patient down from the refusal to get in the shower or attempt to reason about how many decades they have spent showering and nothing bad ever happened. You are up against a wall of fear and you have to find a way over it. If you are still doing all the caregiving tasks yourself, with no outside help, this is a really good time to change that.

I know there may be financial constraints, but if you can just arrange to have a helper come for short stints and handle the bathing and dressing, you will be doing yourself an enormous favor. In all probability, your loved one is not going to fight an outside person as hard as they fight you. You have a history with them, you have pushed each other's buttons in the past, and you still know how to do it. You should not be the one trying to bathe your parent, your spouse, or your partner. This is especially true if it's a parent with whom you have had a challenging relationship. Bathing them is too intimate, too loaded, and it's going to be the setup for a fight that you don't want to have.

This subject often brought out some defensiveness in members of the support group. Someone would point out that a friend whose mother had cancer bathed her when she was too weak from chemo to do it herself, and no problems arose. Someone else would float the idea that the intimacy of bathing is exactly why the family member should be the one to do it. But dementia is a different world from cancer, with a different logic: most of the time there isn't any logic. There is chaos and unpredictability. There are tantrums and behavioral changes that can give you whiplash.

It's obviously an individual choice as far as how hands-on you want to be, but I've heard enough stories and seen enough tears to know that there are certain things that are best left to a trained caregiver who is not related to your loved one. Taking on the most intimate aspects of caregiving is overwhelming. Your days will be spent trying to figure out how to get your loved one bathed and dressed, and you will be exhausted.

ALL THIS BEING SAID, let's move to the mechanics of getting bath time to proceed smoothly, no matter who takes on the task. First, try getting a handheld shower nozzle and a shower chair; any medical supply company will have seats with a back so the person sitting is in no danger of tipping backward. Try bathing your loved one without letting the water come down on top of them, which the handheld device will permit. If the fear is centered around the water coming down, this may work. If the fear comes from somewhere else, you'll know right away.

If the new way of showering doesn't work, you're going to have to try using a tub. Once the person is in the tub, replace the handheld nozzle with a washcloth. Tubs have their challenges, as it's easy for someone to slip getting in and out. This is another reason to have outside help. Trained caregivers know how to get a person in and out of a tub safely.

I learned from cofacilitators in my support group the importance of timing and setting the mood for bathing. Make a specific time of the day bath time. Typically, people with Alzheimer's start to sleep later and later in the morning, so pick a time in the afternoon and stick to it. Even if they don't know what time it is, a biological rhythm is still operating. If three o'clock is predictably bath time, they will sense that. And if you still get resistance, go to every other day, but stick to the established time.

Setting the mood can make a big difference. One idea is to play music, whatever music your loved one likes. Make sure it's the same music each day. And have something comfortable ready for them after the bath, like a soft robe that will feel good and (hopefully) distract from whatever was upsetting about bathing. Try scented oils like lavender, which is calming, although most dementia patients have a poor sense of smell. Avoid scented candles for the obvious reason that they pose a fire danger.

I know many cases where these kinds of ritual worked. The dementia patient got caught up, transported by the music, and forgot what was previously upsetting about water, or looked forward to the feel of a soft wrap, or knew that a particular hour of day was bath time, and could focus on that. Such routine seems to keep fears at bay. But not everyone is so lucky. Dementia patients can surprise you with what they remember. You might think they'll forget whatever was scaring them about bathing, only to find out that the fear doesn't go anywhere.

If none of these methods work, you will have to resort to sponge baths, maybe even just with adult wipes. Just don't give up. Poor hygiene results in a myriad of health issues including bacterial infections, bladder infections that can move up to the kidneys, and skin problems. Urinary-tract infections are the most common result of insufficient bathing and, while these are more common in women, men can also get them. Be aware of a symptom that is not usually associated with UTIs: in elderly people with dementia, a UTI frequently presents as a sharp, rapid decline in cognitive abilities. The patient can become extremely irrational, even delusional. Often caretakers assume that the dementia has plummeted to a new level, but it's worth taking your loved one for a checkup, particularly if the change comes on suddenly. They can't tell you about their discomfort or their physical symptoms; depending on how the synapses in their brain are functioning, they might not even be aware of their own physical symptoms. In many cases, what seems like a massive change in someone's mental capacity may turn out to be a UTI, and once the person is put on antibiotics, they return to the functional level they were at before. Obviously, the best scenario is to try to avoid an infection like this, so the importance of bathing can't be ignored.

✑

DENTAL HYGIENE CAN BE another problem, although generally it doesn't seem to give rise to the same hysteria as bathing. Problems in this area seem to have more to do with confusion. My mother told me during the early stages of my father's Alzheimer's that he no longer understood how to use the Waterpik. (My parents were early Waterpik converts; they used it religiously every night and touted their improved dental checkups.) Suddenly my father was baffled by the device. Wisely, my mother didn't push it. In the late stages of the disease, when he was bedridden, he didn't understand spitting out the water and toothpaste, so the nurses wiped his teeth with paper towels wet with a small amount of toothpaste.

When we need our teeth cleaned or worked on, we go to a dentist's office. This can be a big issue for someone with dementia. It's a different place, there are instruments, noises, a dentist's fingers in their mouth, and commands they may not understand. The good news is that there are dentists who specialize in treating people with dementia. And there are also, in some areas, mobile dentists who will come to the home. I suggest having X-rays done in the early stages of the disease, so the dentist has a baseline, because in the latter stages getting X-rays may be difficult. It's vital to remember that someone with dementia may be in pain and not able to tell you.

My family learned a similar lesson one year when a particularly bad flu was going around; everyone in my parents' house got it, despite their flu shots. I got sick as well, so I was not visiting, but my mother described to me how confused my father seemed by his symptoms. He was obviously in distress but couldn't communicate what the specific causes were. We concluded that he must have had no memory of being sick with the flu in the past, so this was all new to him. I could only imagine how scary it must have been to feel horrible and have no understanding of what was going on. I wish I could tell you that we found some effective method of explaining it to him but, sadly, we couldn't think of anything to do. It was one of our most helpless feelings during those years, watching him suffer with symptoms he couldn't comprehend or describe.

TYPICALLY, ELDERLY PEOPLE WHO are diagnosed with any kind of dementia probably have at least one other physical ailment for which they are taking medication. It's really important to get their medications away from them and give them what they need at the appropriate times. Near-fatal episodes can occur when someone with dementia gets medications mixed up and overdoses on something meant to be taken once a week. In the early stages of Alzheimer's you can try using those pill boxes marked with the days of the week to organize the medications for each week. But keep a close watch. It's just too easy for someone even in the early stages of dementia to make a mistake.

Changing medication procedures is one of those difficult transitions, like taking away the car or changing the bathing ritual. People tend to feel very proprietary about their medications and their ability to self-administer them. To the person with dementia, it probably feels infantilizing to have the responsibility taken away. To get beyond that, try personalizing the process: tell them that you also get confused with medications, get a pill organizer for yourself, and explain that you need the reminders of which pill to take when. Even if you don't take any medications, invent a story and have props to back it up. Use vitamins or over-the-counter pills to fill up your box.

Once you do get your loved one's medications away from them, hide the pills. Just as children seem to unearth things you've hidden away, so do people with Alzheimer's. They are going to know, at least for a while, that something was taken from them, and they will go looking for it.

Be mindful that with medications people's body chemistry changes; their tolerance for a drug they have been on for years alters as they get older and, it seems, as a disease like Alzheimer's takes over. Your loved one could have a reaction to drugs they have taken for decades and be unable to tell you. It's difficult to get someone with Alzheimer's to the doctor's office for a blood test, but if you combine that with something they enjoy—a drive down to the beach or a walk, a lunch outing if they are still able to do that—then going for the blood test will just be one component of an otherwise nice day.

☙

THESE CONSIDERATIONS ARE SOME of the most humbling aspects of dementia—the flesh-and-bone realities of being human. When the disease first enters our lives, we don't think about having to deal with bathing issues and teeth cleaning; we are focused on our loved one's mental decline and the way their emotions shred and fall apart. We are thinking about our own loss, our sorrow, and sometimes about the complexity of our relationship with the person who is ill. But as the disease progresses, we're brought down to the most basic human needs. We are witness to the helplessness that takes over on a physical level, and it's a new pain mixed with embarrassment and discomfort.

Many of us think we can tackle any challenge that comes our way, but it's important to accept that at times the best thing we can do for ourselves is take a step back and let someone else handle things. That's why I have emphasized that you should not be the one tending to intimate activities like bathing. If financial constraints prohibit getting an outside caregiver, you can get respite care, where a helper will come in temporarily for shorter periods of time. Respite care is widely available and was started for people who could not afford outside caregivers on a regular basis.

The main point here is that you need to care for yourself too, and for your own grieving process. Dealing with the awkwardness and the uncomfortable emotions of bathing your parent, dressing them as you would a child, is not going to help you with your grief, it's going to get in the way. There will be moments, no matter what you do, when you are going to witness the physical frailty of your loved one, and it will hurt in a different way than watching their mental decline. These are profound moments and they need to be acknowledged and revered. But the healthiest thing you can do is impose some boundaries on what you're asking of yourself.

My family was very fortunate to be able to hire an outside caregiver fairly early in my father's disease. The man who tended to him in the early days was gentle and soft-spoken, and when it was clear that my father shouldn't go into the shower unattended, it was not a dramatic turn of events. I didn't witness it, but my mother told me that there was a new way of doing things and my father had accepted it.

I remember the moment when it hit me that my father was now frail, weakened by age and Alzheimer's. I was walking with him and his caregiver down the hallway in my parents' house. There were windows along one side of the hall, and afternoon sun was moving lower in the sky, splintering between leaves and tree branches as it came through the glass. Suddenly my father stopped, bent down slowly, and got on his knees. He began rubbing a spot on the floor as if trying to wipe something away. I realized that he thought the freckles of sunlight shining on the floor were something that had spilled and he was trying to clean it up. We helped him to his feet and tried to explain that it was just sunlight. I'm not sure he understood, but the moment passed for him. Except for me, it didn't. Seeing him kneeling on the floor like that hit me in the gut. He looked so narrow and thin, so different from the strong, sturdy man I had gazed up at as a child, the man I thought could do anything. His hands were pale and almost translucent as he tried to mop up pieces of sunlight. I was acutely aware that I was feeling a different kind of heartbreak—the rawness of seeing how a body diminishes as life nears its end. It frightened me, and as much as I knew I had to own the feeling, I also wanted to balance it with something less terrifying.

I thought about the story a nurse told after my father was shot and was recovering in the hospital. She came into his room and found him kneeling on the floor, mopping up some water he had spilled. He told her he didn't want anyone else to have to clean it up since he had spilled it. This was who he was, I thought—a man who didn't want anyone to be inconvenienced by a small mess he had made, a man who tried to wipe spots of sunlight off the floor.

"Let everything happen to you. Beauty and terror. Just keep going. No feeling is final."   —RAINER MARIA RILKE

CHAPTER 14

The Hardest Decision

Varying degrees of difficulty attend the decision to put your loved one in a facility, but I have not met anyone who came to it lightly. It's a decision that, once made, is basically permanent, and it's a grim marker in the course of the disease. For my friends Cara and Thomas, long-time attendees of my support group, it was incredibly hard to decide to put Cara's mother, Michelle, into a full-time facility. Even long after they knew that they had made the right decision, guilt still crept up on them.

It is always helpful to go to the root of any emotion. When the subject of placing your loved one in a facility comes up, the feeling of guilt is fueled by the fear that you might be abandoning them. So, let's tackle that first. Abandoning someone is driving them out to the Mojave Desert, tossing them out of the car, and leaving them there. Or some other version of that scenario. Placing your loved one in a facility where they will get round-the-clock care, where there is little or no risk of them wandering off, where there is a dependable structure to each day as well as activities that might stimulate and entertain them is not abandonment, it's responsible care. There comes a point in this disease when—for most people—caring for a dementia patient at home is just not sustainable. For one thing, it's very expensive. I know roughly the cost of my father's home care, and it was exorbitant. It was, fortunately, a cost my parents could bear; moreover, because my father had been president and there were always security concerns, the question of whether to place him somewhere else was never even introduced.

One of the things that makes the decision so hard, and a reason people want to avoid it, is that it's another milestone. And the situation of waiting for an opening at a nursing home brings you face to face with death. A place only opens up when someone dies. It's another reminder that you have no control over this disease. Whichever way you turn, a shadow waits patiently, a shadow that will come for all of us someday. We all have trouble facing it.

In the late nineties, when I started lecturing about my experience of losing a parent to Alzheimer's, I became familiar with the world of nursing homes and dementia-care facilities. I toured a few facilities during that time. Even though that scenario wasn't a reality for my family, I was acutely aware that we were in the minority, and that many families had to weigh whether or not to put their loved one into a home and, if so, which one would be the best. Years later, when I began my support group, this subject came up practically every week. It's daunting, and there is no one-size-fits-all answer.

As I write this, horror stories about nursing homes are prominent in the news. With the coronavirus pandemic, massive deaths have occurred in nursing facilities around the country. Some of these places did the best they could—they are, after all, contained environments where any virus that gets in is likely to sweep through and infect an already vulnerable group of residents. But some facilities were grossly irresponsible. In one elder-care home in New Jersey seventeen bodies were piled up in a back room.[5] The Center for Medicare and Medicaid Services now requires all nursing facilities to report any Covid-19 cases to the Centers for Disease Control and Prevention (CDC).

As horrible as the effects of the pandemic are, it can't be an excuse for people to decide not to place their loved ones in a facility when it's clear that their current living situation is no longer working. It is unfortunately going to be yet another thing that you have to investigate, but there should be clear records of what facilities were affected by Covid-19 and how they handled it. The handling really should be where your judgment comes in, not whether or not the virus showed up there, as we know now that the virus is insidious and highly contagious. But look carefully at the information available: some facilities that did not handle the crisis responsibly have changed ownership and management.

❧

NO MATTER HOW METHODICALLY you try to prepare for what dementia will bring into your life, it is inevitable that the disease will surprise you. Your parent, or spouse, or relative might still be somewhat functional on Monday, then on Friday be completely disoriented and incapable of remembering anything. Sometimes there have been signs along the way that you didn't notice—warnings that slipped past you. Sometimes the disease just makes a quantum leap into the next stage. And sometimes some family members notice things changing while others don't.

A man who brought his mother into his home to live with him and his family is certain this is the best choice. His wife and teenage kids go along with his decision, and at first it isn't too disruptive. The mother has been diagnosed with Mild Cognitive Impairment, which means that most of the time she is functional and can interact with everyone, including the teenagers. She can help out in the kitchen, carry on conversations about current events; she spends time out in the garden reading.

But the man goes to work every day, and the kids go to school. The wife is left caring for her mother-in-law; she is the one who witnesses the decline of cognition, the memory gaps that grow more frequent. She's the one who has to keep an eye on an elderly woman who now can't really be trusted in the kitchen and who might wander off at any moment. It's upending life as she once knew it. When she tries to talk to her husband about it, he's tired after work, and doesn't really want to hear it. His denial is not only about his mother, it's also about the fact that his marriage is fraying. His wife is exhausted, stressed, and feels it's unfair that she has been thrust into the role of primary caregiver for her mother-in-law without ever being asked if that was okay with her.

The situation erupts when the man's mother walks out the back door while her daughter-in-law is upstairs. By the time her absence is noticed, enough time has passed that she could be anywhere. The police are called, an alert is put out for a woman with dementia who is lost, and she is finally found sitting by the edge of a busy four-lane highway. Thankfully, she's unhurt, but the fractures that have opened up in this family will take time and work to heal, and there is no certainty that they can be healed.

Placing the man's mother in a facility is a subject that should have been discussed long before things got to the breaking point. It's not an easy conversation, but the cost of not putting it on the table and at least talking about it is high. Marriages can suffer, resentments can fester, and it's possible these problems may never go away.

✌☩

A WOMAN WHOSE MOTHER will not move from her condo and barely allows an outside caregiver in, agreeing to only a few hours a week, is becoming more and more forgetful. But she remembers that her daughter once promised her that she would never be moved out of her home. Her daughter, an only child, can't find the stamina to stand up to her mother. Her father died many years ago and it's been a family of two for a very long time, with her mother the dominant force.

Then one day, another resident at the condominium contacts her. Her mother has been pounding on neighbors' doors at all hours of the day and night, sometimes in her nightgown. The neighbor says that if this continues, she will have no choice but to call either the police or Adult Protective Services, or both. So, the uncomfortable process of a daughter shifting the balance and taking control of her mother's life—a process that should have evolved over a period of time—has to be accomplished at lightning speed. This woman is now faced with the reality of finding an appropriate facility, insisting that her mother must move, and somehow getting caregivers into the condo in the meantime so that her mother's behavior can be controlled and the authorities aren't notified. It's like a hurricane slamming into one's life versus a slow-moving storm where there is time to make the necessary decisions.

And consider this: many facilities have a waiting list. It's not as though you can make a decision and, a week later, start the process of moving your loved one in. I know people who have had to wait four or five months before there was an opening in the chosen facility.

There is nothing easy about this decision. It's particularly hard if you don't have any other family members and are the sole caregiver. This is a time when you really need someone you can talk to, but it's also a time when you need to be discerning about whom you choose to confide in. A support group is the best choice, but if you can't find one, seek out a friend who has had some experience with dementia, someone who is less inclined to judge and hold to preconceived opinions. Feelings about nursing facilities can be strong, and a person who has no personal experience with how wrenching a decision this is may have opinions that are unreasonable. This is not someone you want to confide in.

I was surprised to discover that I had some judgments on the subject during the earlier years of my father's illness. My mother had a friend whose husband also had Alzheimer's. They were very wealthy, and she had round-the-clock caregivers for her husband. So it seemed odd to me that she decided to place her husband in a home. My mother gave me no details, she simply told me that this was going to happen. Her friend placed her husband fairly quickly, and a week later he died. I found myself thinking that if she had left him home with the caregivers she already had, he might have lived longer. I had never met this man, but I allowed myself to bend into ideas like, "He probably died from heartbreak at having been taken from his home."

I was uncomfortable with where my mind was going. I realized that I had no idea how Alzheimer's had manifested in this man; I didn't know what the home situation was or how difficult things might have been for my mother's friend or for the caregivers. I was deeply ashamed that I had veered into such a critical attitude, but I'm glad in retrospect that this happened. Years later, when I started Beyond Alzheimer's, one of the ground rules that I was adamant about was not judging others.

While there are points of similarity among Alzheimer's cases, the disease is different in every person it claims. My mother's friend might have been dealing with an impossible situation that couldn't be controlled by round-the-clock caregivers. I just don't know. No one has a right to sit in judgment of the decisions people make regarding their loved one's care, with the obvious exception of clear-cut neglect or abuse.

❧

ONCE THE DECISION IS made to look for a suitable facility, then comes the daunting task of finding the right one. One thing you might want to remember is that *you* are not going to be living there. That sounds obvious, but I have listened to people tell me that they ruled out one facility because it was "so depressing," with elderly Alzheimer's residents sitting around not doing much and clearly not knowing who they were talking to, if they were in fact talking to another person and not just the air. If you don't like the color of the walls or think the lino-leum floors are outdated and tacky—remember that you are not going to be moving in. Your aesthetics cannot be the determining factor.

You have choices as to the type of facility. Small nursing homes house only six or eight people: the ratio of nurses to patients is bet-ter in these small boutique facilities, but the patients may not get organized activities like music or movies. Larger facilities generally do have more activities, but you should find out exactly how they attempt to stimulate and entertain the residents. Many larger facilities have a three-tiered system. Individuals who are still able to function well on their own can go into the assisted-living section; when their dementia gets worse, they can be moved into the skilled nursing section. The third area, for when the late stages of dementia have closed in, is memory care. The advantage of this tiered system is that when your loved one gets worse, they don't have to physically move to a completely different facility.

Researching all of this can feel like falling down a rabbit hole. But think about how things were decades ago, when there weren't really any choices when it came to nursing facilities. My grandmother, Nelle Reagan, who had some form of dementia (diagnoses were not very good then, and memory loss was referred to as senility) spent her last days in a large room with many other patients, all lying in cots, the stale air heavy around them. So it's something to be grateful for that we have progressed to trying to create restful environments at the last stage of life for those who are ill and unable to care for themselves. As burdensome as it is to make the right choice for placing your loved one, you do have choices.

A friend of mine whose mother had Alzheimer's came up with an innovative way of choosing a facility when the inevitable time came. She would show up unannounced during lunchtime. If the place was too quiet, if the residents were sitting there silently spooning food into their mouths, she would assume they were probably all medicated, and she would cross that place off her list. When she finally walked into a facility that was noisy and hectic during lunchtime, with residents talking over each other, some complaining, some laughing, some talking to themselves, she knew that was the right place for her mother. She was right—her mother adjusted quickly and was happy there for the remainder of her days.

Other people I know, whose loved ones were in earlier stages of dementia, took them to a facility for lunch without telling them what the place was to gauge their reactions, see if they seemed comfortable or were uneasy. It's not a perfect method, since dementia can have ups and downs for reasons that elude the caregivers, but it's a reasonable test. If that's not workable, someone from the facility may make a home visit to meet your loved one, not announcing that they come from a nursing facility.

Questions to ask about nursing facilities include the ratio of attendants to residents, as well as how the days and evenings are structured. When are mealtimes? When is there some form of activity, even if it's just drawing or singing? Ask whether the program incorporates music sessions for the residents. Is there a set schedule when a doctor comes to check the residents, or is a doctor only called when there is an obvious health issue? Nursing facilities are not cheap, so, to be blunt, you want to know what you are paying for. And you want to have an idea of what your loved one's days are going to look like.

Recently I heard about a facility with a completely different approach. It does not structure the day, does not establish set times for meals. Instead, it lets the residents do whatever they want, whenever they want, and it claims that everyone is happier this way. I try to be open-minded, but this sounds like complete chaos to me. In fact, when I first learned about it, I had an instant image of Romper Room with elderly people in various stages of dementia. In my view, one of the advantages of placing a loved one in a facility is that there is a structure that the residents come to rely on, even if they don't cognitively understand it. They can sense that it's nearing the lunch hour or the dinner hour. Their days settle into a rhythm that is grounding and dependable. If lunch is always at noon, at 11:45 they will almost certainly start to feel hungry. Chaos and Alzheimer's are not a good combination.

Most reputable facilities offer music sessions when the residents can sing together or listen to someone play the piano or another instrument. Many studies have been done on how music affects dementia patients: it's undisputed that music seems to have a therapeutic effect, grounding them, even making them a little less volatile. But why some patients remember music when they can't recall other things is a mystery. When my father still attended church, in the early stages of the disease, his cognition and memory were noticeably affected, yet he could sing church hymns from memory. In the Glen Campbell film *I'll Be Me*, we are allowed to witness the unraveling of Campbell's thought process and the withering of his memory, but when he picks up a guitar or banjo, he doesn't miss a note. This sort of memory retention doesn't happen with everyone, and it may be a mystery that's never solved, but music remains a valuable therapeutic tool.

✵

ONCE YOU'VE SELECTED a facility, you have the challenge of how to move your loved one in with as little drama as possible. Most reputable facilities provide someone who will assist you with this—advise you, coordinate things on their end. It can require an immense amount of strategy and subterfuge to accomplish the move. Someone with Alzheimer's might not know what day it is, or what they had for breakfast, but they will know if they're being moved out of their home. The decision that brought you here was hard. Carrying it out is going to be harder.

You will want to include many personal items—photos, bedding, even some small pieces of furniture—so that your loved one's new home has a familiarity to it. This is challenging because the space should be ready when the patient gets there, but you don't want to telegraph ahead of time that something is changing. What's worked for many people is to plan something else first, like a lunch or an outing, on the day of the move, to get the person out of the home they are leaving. While you do that, others can transport the items you've selected to the facility.

Among the items to take are photographs and scrapbooks, important for someone with Alzheimer's. Their short-term memory isn't functioning because the synapses in the brain aren't firing properly. And many parts of their long-term memory fall away. But what usually remains are the memories with deep roots, the memories that have encoded themselves in their brains, and they are vivid. Photos can help trigger those memories and ground the person in a time frame that feels real. It's not just that they are recollecting what happened: it's as if they are there again. When my father saw a football game on television and believed that it was his college team and he needed to get out there on the field, it was absolutely real to him. He remembered some of the names of his teammates; he said something about the rain having stopped so the game was on. The woman who sees a photo of herself as a child with her parents is there again on that Easter Sunday, with bees buzzing across the field where Easter eggs were hidden, with her crinoline dress scratching her and making her uncomfortable. A man who travels back to a time when he played catch with his father in the backyard feels again the smack of the ball against his leather glove, feels the late spring air brushing past him, and inhales the smell of blooming jasmine. Photographs can give your loved one someplace to go; they can linger there, rest in the familiarity of the images, hear again voices they once relied on, and revisit a world that may be gone, but has come back to make them feel at home for a while.

One day in the last year of my father's life I slipped a photograph into my pocket when I went to visit him. It showed him as a young lifeguard in his bathing suit, standing near the river where he spent his summers. My father was still awake for much of the day then, but he had stopped speaking. When we were left alone, I showed him the picture. His eyes lingered on it, focused, and then he looked straight at me, holding my gaze for several minutes. I saw behind his eyes the river's currents, felt how they are warmer on top and colder the farther down you plunge. I imagined how the water pulled against his arms with each stroke as he swam, slapped at his feet as he kicked hard across the surface, whether for exercise or to reach someone who was drowning. I thought of Norman Maclean's line in his novel *A River Runs Through It*: "Eventually, all things merge into one, and a river runs through it." The image in the photograph allowed my father to return to those summers, to the river he loved, the river that never stopped running through his life.

There are pieces of the past that Alzheimer's leaves alone, like open windows the disease has passed by, not bothering to close them. If you can direct your loved one to one of those windows, you will be giving them a gift that can't be equaled in the narrow world of their present-day life.

⁂

ONCE YOU GET YOUR loved one to the facility where, hopefully, their new space is ready, the moment of truth has arrived. I don't believe that lying or altering reality is your best choice at this point. Even if they don't fully understand what you're saying, it's best to tell them as clearly and succinctly as you can that this is now going to be home, and you will visit often. It will be a better, safer place, and they will make new friends and be well cared for. Don't mention that you won't be visiting for a couple of weeks: any reputable facility will counsel you to stay away for approximately two weeks, so that your loved one can acclimate. If you keep showing up during this transition period, the limbo state will persist, generated by the desire to return to the home they know while at the same time they are being inundated with new images and faces. You want them to shift into an acceptance of this new place as their home. And they will, but it will happen more easily if you get out of the way for a bit. It may be rocky at first, and there may be hysterics occasionally. But remember that for someone with Alzheimer's things move quickly, including their reasons for being upset. Obviously, some people adjust more quickly than others, but generally two weeks is enough for this new reality to fold around them and for them to relate to it as home, or at least a version of home.

Unfortunately, no matter how you prepare yourself, or counsel yourself, there will probably still be times when you question your decision. My friend Cara said that long after her mother was settled and content in her new home, she would still have moments of asking herself if she did the right thing. This is when getting past guilt is really a herculean effort.

If you were very close to your parent, as Cara was with her mother, guilt is going to be threaded into the fact that you miss that parent. Your devotion to them sends you down a path of thinking that maybe you should have sacrificed the quality of your own life just to keep them in the place they were accustomed to. It's going to be a persistent battle of emotion versus reality. The truth is, your parent is better off in a place where there is constant and professional care, a dependable structure to the days, and a low risk of getting lost or setting the place on fire.

❧

IT'S PARTICULARLY WRENCHING WHEN you have to place your spouse or partner in a facility. Marriage vows state "in sickness and in health." People wonder "Doesn't that mean I should have kept them with me no matter what?" No. It means you need to consider the reality of what's going on and make the most responsible decision for your loved one and for yourself. In this circumstance, you will be left with the emptiness in your home, your bed, at the breakfast table, on Saturdays when you had a standing reservation for "date night." And within that emptiness, thoughts will pull at you, haunt you, make you wonder if you did the right thing.

A woman I know made the decision to place her husband in a facility and then started to doubt her decision. After a few weeks, she took her husband out and brought him home. It did not work out well. He was confused, agitated, even angry, and she realized she'd made a disastrous choice. She took her husband back to the facility (fortunately they still had room for him) and he had to get oriented all over again. I wish I could offer some formula for making the transition easier, more bearable, but I can't. The doubts will settle down, the thoughts that scream at you will soften, but it will take some time. Just as your loved one has to adjust to a new home, so do you.

❧

MANY ALZHEIMER'S PATIENTS TALK about home—whether they are in their own home, a family member's home, or a facility. "I want to go home" is a phrase that countless caregivers have heard. It can be confusing and distressing if the person uttering those words is in their own home. Do they mean their childhood home? Do they mean the dorm room they lived in when they went to college? Their first apartment? People have told me that they tried to show their loved one that they were still home by pointing out all the familiar items in a room or reminiscing about Thanksgiving dinners in the dining room. And still the phrase is repeated: "I want to go home."

This is what I've come to believe, and there is obviously no medical basis for it, but it makes sense to me. I think when dementia patients say this, they are talking more about a feeling than an actual place. Imagine what it must be like to have everything become increasingly fragmented, whittled away. Your landscape is always changing, shifting; you see faces that look familiar, but you can't place who they are. It must be the most disorienting feeling, as though you have been dropped into a foreign land and you can't get your bearings. Home is not just a place, it's a feeling inside us—a sense that we are anchored somewhere, that we belong, where we know what is around the next corner. That we are safe. Alzheimer's patients have none of that. They are unmoored, adrift, and tomorrow might be even more uncertain than today.

What I have suggested is that people talk to their loved one about the family members and friends who care about them and are around them. That's what home is—the love of those who care about you and are there for you. Let them know that no matter where they are physically, they will always be home because that embrace of love will be there for them. I am not suggesting that this will produce a miracle—your loved one might still say, "I want to go home." But because I believe that the soul hears and understands everything on a deep, invisible plane, those words might get through and make a difference, even if it doesn't seem so at the moment.

When my friends Cara and Thomas visited Michelle in the facility that became her home, they brought her pictures of their son's new baby. They told her that she was a great-grandmother and shared cute stories about the baby. Michelle would light up and drink in every word. The next time they came and showed her a picture, it was all new to her again. She had no memory of being told before that this was her great-grandchild, but each time she was filled with love and joy. Each time she was reminded that she was home.

So many things at this stage pulse with reminders that the end is moving closer. Your head argues with your heart. You know that your loved one is being cared for by people who are trained for this, you know that your visits are easier now because you aren't worried about what kind of trouble your loved one might get into, or what disaster might be waiting around the bend—are we sure they didn't turn the stove on or try to get on the computer? Are we sure we put detergent and cleansers out of reach? You don't have those worries, yet your heart hurts. This disease is like crossing a mountain range. There are easy trails, downward slopes, and there are steep climbs that feel impossible. The point is to keep going and to find people to help you along the way.

"You return to that earlier time armed with the present, and no matter how dark that world was, you do not leave it unlit."

—MICHAEL ONDAATJE, *Warlight*

REBUILDING YOUR WORLD

CHAPTER 15

The World They Have Created

In 2007, Sandra Day O'Connor revealed through a family member that her husband, who was in the late stages of Alzheimer's and was in a facility, had fallen in love with another resident there.[1] John O'Connor had no memory of the life he had lived with his wife and children; in the longing for connection, he began a new relationship. When his wife visited, she saw them sitting outside on a bench, holding hands. The reason for releasing this information was to say publicly that she was happy for him. She was grateful that he was content and had companionship in his life. I remember that when that story came out, I was so moved that she had the courage to say to the world that this was what Alzheimer's does—it erases memory, but it doesn't erase desire for other people.

This is a dramatic example of what love is supposed to be. Sandra Day O'Connor didn't get mired in jealousy or resentment, nor was she sidelined into feeling like a victim. She loved her husband—in sickness and in health—which meant his happiness was her happiness. She still visited him, watched him with his new partner, and rested in the knowledge that, with so much having been stolen from him by Alzheimer's, including his history with her, he found someone to fill that empty space.

Justice O'Connor had resigned from the Supreme Court a year earlier to care for her husband. She then came to the sad realization that he would be better off in a facility with trained people who knew more about Alzheimer's than she did. Her openness in revealing the details of what she has gone through has helped countless people. In 2013, she once again let us into her private world, revealing that she too had been diagnosed with Alzheimer's.

I believe that by being open about her husband's new partner, and her wise response to that situation, O'Connor taught the world a valuable lesson about love, understanding, and kindness. She also opened a window into the world of Alzheimer's and let us see what often happens when people forget the life they have lived. This disease can't steal the need for companionship. It's a primal desire that transcends illness. And if the connections and relationships of a lifetime have been erased from memory, a person will seek new ones. People with dementia feel loneliness even if they can't express it, and they want to fill that void.

꿈

DURING THE CORONAVIRUS PANDEMIC I have thought a lot about connections with other people. Most of us have. We find ourselves isolated, either with our families or, if we are alone, with our own thoughts and worries. We are hungry for the camaraderie of other people, for the physical sensation of someone embracing us, or even just standing closer than six feet. Every time we veer away from each other on a sidewalk while we're walking our dog, putting distance between us, it reinforces the sad reality that we can't connect right now—not the way we used to, anyway. And we all harbor the same fear that we may never be able to connect in the same way again. I've seen the concern in people's eyes as they move away quickly, and I suspect the same is visible in mine. It's reminded me more than once of what I saw in my father's eyes in the early stages of Alzheimer's. He would sometimes gaze at the room he was in, or the people around him, with a look of muted desperation, as if he wanted to connect with something or someone familiar to him, but everything was splintering, turning into a foreign land. I even saw it sometimes when he looked at my mother, although I would never have mentioned that to her.

Mother Teresa said, "The most terrible poverty is loneliness, and the feeling of being unloved." If the people in one's life become unrecognizable, if the relationships that anchored them through decades fade into the fog of Alzheimer's, essentially disappearing, the loneliness must be unbearable. Even more so because the person who is experiencing that loss can't communicate it.

So, for someone with Alzheimer's, who feels distance yawning around them, who sees faces that should be recognizable but aren't, who wanders through rooms that no longer feel like home, the only companion left is fear. If they are placed into a living situation with other people, whose eyes match theirs, whose arms reach for them, they are going to grab on and not let go, because suddenly fear has moved aside and there is a hand to hold, a body next to theirs that fits with their new version of home.

❧

IT'S ACTUALLY A VERY common occurrence for people with dementia who have been placed in facilities to start up relationships.[2]

It's sometimes puzzling for others who hear about this because the assumption is that Alzheimer's patients are elderly and the desire for romance must have dwindled long ago. But dementia moves a person back through time, so in the mind of someone with Alzheimer's, they are not eighty or ninety—they might be twenty, or even sixteen. I have heard of several instances when an elderly person with Alzheimer's complained about the facility they had been moved into because "there are so many old people here."

In one situation a woman became smitten with another resident at a facility, believing he was her college sweetheart. She called the man by that boy's name, and the man went along with it. They convinced each other that they had gone on dates recently, dined at restaurants, taken moonlit walks. They created a new world for themselves in which they were happy, in love, and young.

I've also heard stories from people who work in nursing facilities about finding residents in each other's rooms, snuggled up in bed together. Some facilities think it best to separate the smitten residents, while others just leave them alone. I'm not sure the separation idea works out very well. Just like teenagers, as soon those in authority move on, the lovers go right back to the bed they've been sharing.

It can be complicated, as a family member and caregiver, to visit your loved one and find him or her entrenched in a world you are no longer a part of. People with Alzheimer's often can't expand their attention to include you in the narrow world they now inhabit. They might be polite to you, but you are just a visitor passing through. This opens up another level of loss and sadness. That's why I think Sandra Day O'Connor's openness about her husband was so important. There is always a choice about how to respond in any situation. You can feel the ache of loss open up in you, but you can choose to honor those feelings while not being trapped by them. You can decide instead to take in the happiness you see in your loved one and be grateful for their contentment.

❧

REBUILDING YOUR OWN WORLD when your spouse or partner has drifted miles away from you, when memories have crumbled on the road behind them, is one of the hardest challenges. A man whose wife was diagnosed with early-onset Alzheimer's spoke eloquently to me about the difficulty of trying to open himself to love again when his wife was in a care facility. His kids had encouraged him to start dating, just to introduce to himself the idea that life could go on. He said it was a herculean effort to open himself to the possibility of a future with someone else. His wife was still everywhere, even though when he sat with her, she seemed to barely know him. It was a surreal balancing act—trying to envision a new, hopeful future while the present was in front of him, stark and full of pain.

Someone else told me that the grief they were experiencing at this latter stage felt like the grief after a death, only their loved one wasn't dead—they were right there, just living in a different time and a different world. They would visit them and be talking to a stranger, except it wasn't a stranger. So much was familiar, yet so much had changed. It takes a strong resolve, but I think the best course is to use the visits with a loved one to briefly step into their world and play whatever role has been assigned to you. If your father thinks you're his parent, go with it. If your mother thinks you're her sibling, then that's who you are for the time that you're visiting. It's quite possible that the next time you visit, your loved one will think you're someone else they have known, so don't get too attached to any one role.

Another thing that might balance out your sorrow is the chance to learn some things about your loved one that you never knew before. Since they have retreated back in time, you are seeing them as they were long before you knew them; if it's your parent, you might even see them as they were before you were born. One man learned that his father, who was successful, driven, and very dictatorial with his children, stuttered as a child and felt insecure and inadequate. It had never been mentioned in his family, but as his father moved back through the decades, that young boy with a speech impediment showed up. It gave the son a reason to soften toward his father, to find forgiveness for how tyrannical he had been.

One woman found out her mother lost a baby before she was born. Suddenly, her eighty-year-old mother was in her twenties, weeping over the loss of a child her daughter had not known about. All she could do was offer comfort and wonder if her mother ever really grieved over the loss all those years ago.

Family secrets can be unveiled as well. I know of a woman who learned that her father cheated on her mother for quite a long while, conducting an affair with one of their friends. Apparently, her mother, who died before her father got Alzheimer's, never found out. It's obviously impossible to know if the story was true or an invention cobbled together in the mists of the disease. But it would be unusual for an entire memory like that to suddenly form with details intact. The woman assumed that her father was revealing the truth. Her parents' perfect marriage was actually not so perfect.

There is no talking Alzheimer's patients back from a world they have retreated to. You might as well visit it with them. It won't lessen your loss, but it will counterbalance it a bit. In some ways, you're coming full circle with a parent who used to play make-believe with you when you were a child. Now it's your turn to play make-believe with them.

I DON'T KNOW WHAT worlds my father drifted into. I wish I did. There were glimpses in the earlier stages of who he was as a boy, as a young man, and I felt that I had gotten to know a bit more about him, this man who had always mystified me. But he grew silent at a certain point; he basically stopped talking except for a few syllables once in a while. Sometimes I saw him moving his hands in a very deliberate way and I tried to figure out if he was reining in a horse or doing ranch work. Maybe he was moving his hands along with something he was talking about in the depths of his mind, beyond his silence. I had only my own imagination to fill in the blank spaces. But wherever he was, he seemed content.

One day when I visited him, not too long before he died, the song "Danny Boy" was running through my head. I had been listening to Eva Cassidy's rendition of it earlier and it had stayed with me, partly because my father used to sing it to me when I was very young. He was, as usual, lying on his back in the elaborate hospital bed that he lived in then, and his eyes were half open. I started singing "Danny Boy" to him very softly, hoping I might see something ignite in his eyes. I didn't, although I did notice the corners of his mouth turn up slightly. But I once again had to grab onto my faith that, deep inside him, he was remembering, and singing along with me. That day the sky billowed with clouds. My father's bed faced the windows, and I wondered if he was looking out at the oak trees and the cloud-filled sky, or if he was too far away in his own world. It's something else I will never know.

When I was about eight or nine, I ran in from the backyard,

found my father behind his desk writing on his note cards, and pulled him outside to the yard. I pointed up to the sky, where thick gray clouds were bumping into each other and a shaft of sunlight was splitting through like a spotlight. "That's God looking through the clouds at us," I told him.

"Maybe," my father said, nodding and getting an amused look in his eyes. "But you know, God doesn't need a window through the clouds to see us. He's always watching over us."

There were times during the Alzheimer's years when I wondered if God was watching or if He had turned away. But with my father in some distant place and his days on the earth growing short, I reminded myself that faith is what you hold onto for dear life when there aren't any signs or whispers, when things seem bleak and you feel yourself edging toward despair. It was a lonely decade for me, in part because my family was so disjointed. I didn't have the constant embrace around me that strongly bonded families do. So, I often saw myself as a lone pilgrim calling out for God. The memories from my childhood, when my father talked to me about God always being present, always listening and watching, were what pulled me back from despair. They had imprinted themselves on me, and in many ways they became my lifeline.

Alzheimer's is a clever thief. It steals a person in so many different ways. Sometimes you're surprised by the absence that confronts you. Sometimes you're taken aback by what has moved into that absence, what has replaced the person you knew. This is particularly true if the person with Alzheimer's turns into a younger version of themselves—someone you never knew—or if long-buried personality traits rise to the surface. You might find yourself constantly thinking you did not see this coming. I think the salve for the wounds that open up is the knowledge that you are getting to know your loved one in ways you might never have before. Of course, that can be either a good thing or a bad thing. But I believe strongly that curiosity can dull the edges of the pain you're feeling.

I often wished my father hadn't slipped into silence. That wish was resurrected when I started the support group Beyond Alzheimer's and heard so many stories about the personality transformations of people's loved ones, and how they got to see facets of them that had been hidden. I will always wonder what I might have learned about my father if he hadn't drifted so far away, if he hadn't settled in a place where he apparently didn't need a voice. So much changed in the years of his illness—both within me and between the two of us. There was a tranquility, even a familiarity and a comfort level, that had not been present before. But in the deepest places, he remained a mystery. Maybe in some way that was his victory over Alzheimer's, that even an overpowering disease couldn't breach the walls of the citadel where he kept much of himself hidden. As a young girl, I rode behind him on horseback, wondering what he was thinking, what was going through his mind as his eyes roamed over hillsides and fields. As a grown woman, I sat at his bedside wondering many of the same things—where was he? Where had the wanderings of his soul taken him? He left me with both gifts and mysteries, and I have to find contentment with that.

"Out beyond ideas of wrongdoing and rightdoing, there is a field. I'll meet you there. When the soul lies down in that grass, the world is too full to talk about."   —RUMI

CHAPTER 16

Other People's Opinions

When your loved one reaches the late stages of dementia, you may be surprised by the number of people who want to share their opinions with you even though you didn't ask for their views. I remember someone in my support group talking about a friend who accused them of being in denial because they weren't correcting their parent when they mistook them for someone else. Instead, they just went along with it. The friend kept insisting, "But this must hurt you. It has to hurt." It was as if the friend wanted them to feel pain. Sadly, that is the agenda of some people—perhaps not consciously, but some part of them is either invested in your sorrow or has written their own script for how they think a story about Alzheimer's should go.

It's often at this point, when caregivers have worked diligently to process what's happening, that other relationships in their life are uprooted. Often in the support group someone who had changed dramatically from the time they first walked in—who had worked hard to accept their grief, who had made the decision to learn from the experience of dementia rather than be a slave to it—had tears in their eyes because a friend had judged them harshly. I have discussed the judgments of others at the early stages of the disease, but that dynamic often becomes more prevalent as decisions have to be made regarding care for a loved one, particularly when placement into a facility is put on the table.

I lost a number of friends in the decade of my father's illness—not so much at the beginning when I was struggling to find my way and my tears were often just beneath the surface, but later, as I began to find my strength. There are people who see it as their prerogative to put you in a particular category. For me, the category I'd been in for a long while was the unhappy girl with a messed-up family, the girl who could never get things right. People felt sorry for me and saw me as predictably and eternally wounded. So, when I began navigating my way through my father's illness, lecturing about what I was learning as the daughter of a man with Alzheimer's—in short, when I began changing and growing—there were people who wanted nothing more to do with me. I had screwed up their filing system. I was no longer in the box they had put me in, and they didn't know where else to put me. It may be trite to say that these are not the kind of people one needs as friends, but it's worth saying because we need to remember it. Real friends are the people who want you to shine.

I had a friend for a long time—through many of my turbulent years—who was a fixture in my life. We were neighbors in California; she was someone I went to for advice and guidance. In fact, that was the dynamic of our relationship: I was the needy one, she was the adult in the room. When I moved back to Los Angeles from New

York, I was already changing. I was being tutored by a disease that had randomly chosen my father, and I was not the same person I had been. I thought my friendship with this woman would resume on my return, and we did see each other, but it was clear to me that something was different. I felt the shift in her attitude toward me. I didn't analyze it too much at that point because I was focused on my father. I told myself I had to accept that she didn't like me anymore, and I tried to move on from the fact that I missed her. I didn't hear from her when my father died. We did see each other once after his death, but it was awkward.

Years passed and I heard from someone that her husband had passed away. I called her a few times and left messages saying how sorry I was and to please let me know if there was anything I could do or if there was anything she needed. I never heard back from her. One morning I was driving home from an early run on the beach and I saw her up ahead on the road, walking with another woman. I pulled over, got out of my car, and, standing in the middle of the street, called out her name. Without slowing down, she glanced over her shoulder, said, "I'll call you, Patti," and kept walking. She never called, nor did I think she would. I remember standing there for a long moment realizing I would never get to embrace her and tell her how sorry I was about her husband; I would never get to ask her how she was holding up or if there was anything I could do to make things easier for her. There is a part of me that will be always be standing on that street, fog brushing past me, watching someone I once called a friend walk away.

It took me a while to analyze what I believe had gone on there. It took hearing the stories of other people who talked about friends leaving them just at the point when they felt they had transformed their lives in such healthy ways. The sad truth is that not everyone will embrace the changes you make in yourself. Every time someone has related a similar story to me, I return to that street and the hollowed out feeling inside me. I wish I had some formula to offer people that would make it easier, but this is one experience you just have to let yourself feel. It helps to understand intellectually how the dynamic changes, what forces are at work, but the abandonment of a friend hurts.

I once went to an open house on a Sunday in my neighborhood. There was a security guard outside because the house was full of possessions. It appeared that nothing had been moved out, including small knick-knacks and framed photographs, and it was fairly evident from the décor that an elderly person lived there. I overheard someone asking the security guard if the owner of the house had passed away (I don't know why they were asking him instead of the real estate agent). The guard rather derisively told the man that the family had moved the woman into a care facility when she got Alzheimer's, and how horrible he thought that was. He made it clear that in his opinion no one should ever be moved out of their own home. I have a bad habit of jumping into situations that don't involve me, and I went over to the security guard and told him that I ran a support group for family members and caregivers of people with Alzheimer's. I asked him if he had ever been around someone with any kind of dementia. He shook his head, no.

"Then maybe you shouldn't judge the decisions family members make. Homes are dangerous places for people with dementia," I told him. "She could have burned the house down, gotten electrocuted, any number of things." I was aware that I was correcting a large man with a gun, but he actually considered what I'd said and agreed that maybe he'd been too hasty with his opinions. Imagine someone close to you leveling that kind of judgment. We can try to dismiss people, ignore what they say, but wounds are still inflicted by ill-chosen words. It's important to remember how tender you are at this stage. If others don't acknowledge that and treat you more gently, then you need to walk away from them.

"What we have once enjoyed we can never lose. All that we love deeply becomes a part of us." —HELEN KELLER

CHAPTER 17

The Empty Seat at the Table

Whether your loved one is in a facility or at home in the late stages of Alzheimer's, it's doubtful they are joining you or other family members at the dinner table. There were times after my father was bedridden when I would go to my parents' house and my mother and I would eat dinner in his room, while a nurse fed him. Other times, if my brother Ron came for a visit, the three of us would eat in the dining room and I felt the weight of the empty chair at the table. It ushered in a flood of memories from long ago, from a time before Alzheimer's—Christmases, my father's cheeks flushed from just a few sips of red wine, or the look on his face when he was about to launch into some serious analysis of America and the world at large. A different look when he was about to tell a funny story. His absence at the table was magnified by the fact that he was just down the hall, lying between white sheets and being fed by a nurse's careful hands.

Years later, I was grateful that I'd felt this wound open up. In my support group were many people who were losing their spouses, and I knew even before I asked that dinner time was particularly hard. It wasn't only romantic dinners they missed, it was the companionship at the end of day, the unraveling of stories about what happened at work, or with the kids, or the next-door neighbor. The dinner table can be its own bubble where you're reminded of what home really means—it's someone who is there when darkness falls, who will listen to you and share with you the details of their day. Without that, loneliness moves in fast and you sink hard into all you've lost.

By the late stages of the disease, someone who is losing a spouse or partner has likely already dealt with the disappearance of their sexual relationship. I'm not suggesting that the loss of intimacy isn't still painful, but there has been time to process it and acclimate to it. The weight of physical absence—the empty side of the bed, the empty chair at the table, the room where they used to work that sits hollow and unused—that weight starts bearing down as dementia slips into its last quiet stages.

During the first few years of my father's illness, my parents ate dinner together as they always had. My mother made a passing comment to me once: "I'm eating dinner with him, but I can't really talk to him anymore," she said. I'm sure that when he couldn't even be physically present at the table her loneliness was worse. Seeing his empty chair there, which no one else ever sat in, allowed me to feel more tenderness toward my mother, one of my biggest challenges during that decade. I didn't lack compassion for her, but it was difficult to feel softness and tenderness when she had never shown the same toward me. So, I grabbed onto the moments when I felt those emotions rise up in me. My father's empty chair at the table was a big one.

I thought about the story of their first date, a dinner date, and how my mother was instantly smitten. I thought of photographs I'd seen of my parents—a glamorous Hollywood couple who were featured in gossip columns and movie magazines, dining at Chasen's, their favorite restaurant. And I thought about the story I was not supposed to know, which I had learned from others. It was over dinner at Chasen's that my mother told my father she was pregnant, and he agreed to marry her. Not the most romantic proposal, which was one reason, among others, that my parents never talked about it. All of that history, all of those emotional seasons, were represented by my father's empty chair at the table.

Left with absence around you, questions drift in that didn't arise before. Like, what if my other parent had gotten Alzheimer's instead? Or, if it's your spouse, what if I had gotten dementia instead of them? How would they be caring for me? A man I know who'd had a very difficult, tormented history with his mother, but a relatively good relationship with his father, watched as his father was consumed by Alzheimer's. He told me something very raw and honest: "Sometimes I feel like the wrong parent got Alzheimer's." He was immediately self-conscious and regretted what he'd said, to the point that tears sprang into his eyes. He said, "That was an ugly thing to say. I'm sorry." But something like that is only ugly if you don't acknowledge that this is not who you want to be. A lot of thoughts come to us that don't reflect who we aim to be as human beings. I think it's important to recognize the thoughts, understand where they come from, so that you can set them aside and not be held hostage by them. Carl Jung believed that if you don't examine the darkness in you—the "shadow self"—it will consume you and define you. What this man said was not the most horrible thing in the world, but it clearly wasn't coming from his more enlightened self, and he recognized that. Jung said, "Everyone carries a shadow, and the less it is embodied in the individual's conscious life, the blacker and denser it is."[3] It's hard to turn a light onto unattractive thoughts and queries, but it's the only way to dispel the darkness of those thoughts.

My inner wanderings didn't go quite as far, but I did wonder sometimes, especially when I sat at the dining table alone with my mother, what it would have been like if Alzheimer's had claimed her instead of my father. What if hers was the empty chair at the table and my father was sitting in his usual spot? Would he have opened up more to his children? Might we have finally gotten to sit with him as a father, not as the parent of America, and forge a relationship with him on a deeper, more personal level? I will never know the answer, of course; it's one more lingering question that will remain forever when I think of my father.

Some people in my support group occasionally filled their lonely dinner hours by going to the facility where their loved one was and having dinner there. I learned from their stories: take your sense of humor along in that situation. You are, after all, dining with a group of residents who are on the dementia spectrum. To say that it will be an unpredictable evening is an understatement. Don't count on eating gourmet food, but that's not really the point. It is, rather, another way to briefly step into your loved one's world while also getting away from the empty chair at your own table. The emptiness will still be there, waiting for you, but you've given yourself a respite.

Another way of looking at this time of loneliness is that it's preparing you for the inevitable end, when your loved one will not be there anymore. You're becoming more familiar with their absence; you're being forced to circle it, get to know it, weigh it against the memories and recollections that have filled up the life you had together. When the end comes, those are the lifelines you will reach for and hang onto.

I often listened from the distance of the dining room to the silence coming from the hallway that led to my father's room. I knew he was there. If I listened hard, I could sometimes hear the nurse's soft voice encouraging him to eat. But mostly it was quiet. I told myself to make friends with that silence because one day, only silence would rest between the walls of that room and trail down the hall. One day he would be gone, and I would again have to hold tightly to my faith and believe that no one is ever really gone, they're just in another place.

"Love knows not its own depth until the hour of separation."

—KHALIL GIBRAN, *The Prophet*

THE END STAGES

CHAPTER 18

Your Old Friend Grief

When I started Beyond Alzheimer's, I educated myself about hospice care. It wasn't something that came up with my father, since he had round-the-clock nurses, but it's important for many people. Hospice and palliative care are different.[1] Palliative care is aimed at improving patients' lives: it includes whatever medications they need and incorporates pain medication as well. Hospice, in contrast, is dedicated to keeping patients comfortable as they are dying. Any life-prolonging medications are removed; pain medications are given as needed.

Every aspect of hospice is palliative—offering comfort—while nothing in basic palliative care constitutes hospice. More precisely, hospice focuses on the last six months of a person's life, after it has been determined that there is no cure and no reason for aggressive therapies. Obviously, in the case of dementia a cure is not yet a relevant concern, but sometimes patients have other health issues that they are being treated for to help keep them alive. With hospice, as I said, those medications are discontinued; only those used to alleviate pain and discomfort are given.

Some people in the support group expressed concern about the six-month time frame of hospice. They worried that if their loved one was still alive after six months, they would no longer be able to have hospice care. That is not the case. They would simply be signed on for another six months, and another and another if it came to that.[2]

Hospice offers many advantages, such as counselors who can speak to family members about the difficult experience of waiting for a loved one to die. The entire agenda is to provide comfort in the last days of life—both for the patient and the family. Morphine is readily available if the person is in pain, especially at the end, on the ledge between life and death.

Hospice as we know it today originated in England with Dame Cicely Saunders, who was initially trained as a nurse but, due to a back injury, gave up nursing.[3] In 1947 she began working as a social worker with seriously ill and dying patients. She observed their suffering, saw how their last days were spent wracked with pain, and decided to dedicate her life to changing how dying people were treated. She became a doctor at the age of thirty-eight. In 1958 she went to St. Joseph's Hospice in the UK, where she researched pain and how—or if—it was being treated. She found that patients were only given morphine sporadically, basically if they were in excruciating pain, and then only by intramuscular injection, which is also painful. Saunders advocated for oral administration of morphine despite resistance in the medical community because doctors feared the patients might become addicted. Let that one sink in—they were worried that dying people in horrible pain might become addicts.

Saunders eventually prevailed and her mission to make the last days of dying patients more comfortable and meaningful began to be realized.

In 1967 Saunders opened St. Christopher's Hospice in South London. It was dedicated to holistic care and was once described as being a combination of "compassion and science."

It's fascinating, yet not surprising, that hospice as we know it today didn't come about easily. Too often, people who are dying are seen as disposable. But Cicely Saunders saw every moment of life, every hour, as being meaningful and important. She died in 2005 at St. Christopher's, surrounded by loved ones and by the peaceful environment she had created. It's easy to take something like hospice care for granted, so it's important to remember it didn't always exist. It took someone with great compassion to decide she was going to change the world in a particular way because it needed to change. Saunders once asked a man who knew he was dying what he needed most of all from those who were caring for him. He said, "For someone to look at me as if they are trying to understand me."

❧

IN *THE TIBETAN BOOK OF LIVING AND DYING*,[4] Sogyal Rinpoche writes poignantly about the challenge of tending to a dying person when in life one's relationship with that person was not ideal: "I have been helped by remembering one thing: that the person in front of me dying is always, somewhere, inherently good." I was struck by that because that's the foundation of forgiveness—seeing in someone else what they have forgotten about themselves. If you believe that we were created by a loving God, then everything that is not loving in us is the result of our own choices, our own free will. That doesn't mean that the soul's beauty isn't still there, it's just buried under a lifetime of rubble and darkness. And, as I said before, if that spiritual view is not something you subscribe to, maybe you could just consider the possibility. It's worth the consideration, especially at the end of someone's life, because it will help you see them as who they were capable of being, rather than just who they chose to be.

No matter the circumstances of a loved one's passing, there is a universal truth about death—the heart looks back and sees everything. It sees the soaring moments of joy, the crippling sorrows, times of anger. It sees betrayals, sacrifices, insecurities, and soul-bending love. In the end people are defined by how their hearts lived. That's also how we will remember our own moments of saying goodbye—how did our hearts choose to embrace the ending of a life that was entwined with ours? I have heard some people say that they deliberately avoided being at the bedside of a loved one—usually a parent—as they were dying. I feel deeply sad for anyone who makes that choice because they miss a profound experience that could stay with them for the rest of their life.

In the deepest ways, the death of a loved one rearranges our own lives, asks us to look at everything and everyone with clear eyes and an open heart. It can rearrange us, shift our priorities and desires, if we let it. Of course, as with all other things, it's a choice. We can turn away and continue as we were, but death is always waiting in some doorway and it will come for all of us when it's ready. It seems wiser to try and make friends with it before that time.

※

AT THE END OF May 2004 it was clear that my father would be gone soon. Swallowing had become difficult, so feeding him any kind of solid food was impossible. Even liquids required patience.

I thought I was prepared for the end. For years I'd felt death hovering—a shadow waiting patiently for the moment it had already decided upon. At certain points it seemed to have moved closer, like when my father had a small stroke (TIA) and we were told this could signal something bigger. Or when the entire household, including my father, caught the flu and the doctor said it might turn into pneumonia. Each time, death reminded me it was there, and I believed I had made friends with it. After all, my father wasn't afraid to die. He had told me all my life that, to him, dying meant going home to God, and how could that be frightening?

But I was about to learn that we are never fully prepared for death. No matter how close it is, or how much we sidle up to it, thinking that familiarity may quell our fears, it always seems to come without warning. The mystery is overwhelming—how can a human being be here one moment and then be gone? Where are they? The existential questions that have plagued mankind for centuries become excruciatingly real. No matter how much you tell yourself beforehand, "I've got this," the truth is you don't.

In Los Angeles, the jacaranda trees were blooming—brilliant purple flowers fell onto sidewalks and streets like lakes of color. Jasmine was blooming too, making the air sultry and sweet. These are the sense memories I have of the time when my father died.

My brother Ron and his wife had gone to Hawaii for their annual vacation. Before they left, Ron came to Los Angeles and as we stood at our father's bedside I said to him, "Are you sure you should be going to Hawaii right now?"

He dismissed the idea that our father might die while he was gone, perhaps because there had been false alarms in the past, or perhaps just because I was the one questioning his judgment. In any event, they went to Hawaii, and less than a week later flew all night to get back in time to say goodbye.

I'll always believe my father waited for Ron. The night before he died it didn't seem as if he would last until morning, although the doctor said it was possible. I left my parents' house when darkness was starting to fall and a full moon was climbing in the sky. I was living in an apartment in a three-unit building and had become close friends with the couple who owned the building, who lived on the ground floor. As I started up the back stairs, which were outside, I suddenly felt I couldn't move. I sat down on the stairs, stared up at the moon overhead, and was overcome with tears. My friends found me there. "I don't know how to lose him," I said. "I don't know how to do this."

They took me inside and we talked for a while—about how no one is ever ready for death, about how it always feels like a surprise even when it really isn't. I will always treasure their companionship at that moment. It brought home to me how universal everyone's experiences of death are, and I remembered that night often years later when death and dying were common subjects in my support group.

When I got to my parents' house just past dawn on June 4, Ron was already there. His plane had landed in the still, dark hours long after midnight and long before dawn. I remember thinking that it's such a lonely time, those hours, and I wondered if he felt their loneliness as he drove from the airport to the hills of Bel Air. But those are conversations that no one in my family ever has, so I didn't ask. We began our vigil at our father's bedside as the sky lightened and fog drifted past the windows. We drank tea, shared memories, and sometimes fell into silence. Instinctively, we kept our voices soft when we spoke, as if we didn't want to disturb our father on his passage out of this world.

At one point, later in the morning, I got up and went outside to the garden. I looked up at the milky sky and felt so many memories and impressions rush in. That's when I realized what a profound teacher death is—it ushers in lessons about life. I had always wished for more of my father, wanting to feel closer to him, to be able to say I had figured out who he was. But even after a decade of seeing layers peeled away, of getting glimpses into him, he was still like paintings in a gallery. There was space between the images, and I had to reconcile myself to the fact that those spaces would forever remain blank.

Through the screen door I could hear my mother in her bedroom talking on the phone. That was basically what she had been doing most of the morning, with the exception of a few times when she came into my father's room. I was suddenly aware that, in the not-too-distant past, I'd have reacted with harsh judgment. Why would she be making phone calls when her children were sitting at their father's bedside, listening to his breathing, waiting for his last exhale? But as the sun started burning away the edges of the fog, I realized that I was not judging her. Instead, I was sad for her. She had no idea how to be part of such an intimate family experience. Neither did my brother and I, but we were doing it—we were reaching past our history and recognizing that this experience needed to transcend everything that had gone before. My mother was missing the gift of sitting with her children as her husband was slowly leaving this earth. It just wasn't in her makeup to participate in that way, and I felt the wrench of heartbreak for her that she had carved out her life in such a way as to miss what was so exquisitely meaningful. I remember saying a silent prayer, thanking death for allowing me to see all of this, for holding up a mirror not only to the past but to the journey I'd taken away from that past.

When the doctor told us that my father's heartbeat was weak and his last breaths were coming, we called my mother in. She was there for the extraordinary moment before my father died, when he opened his eyes—eyes that were blue again, and focused. She got confirmation of his love when he turned his gaze on her just before his final breath. I was happy for her that she got the moment she longed for, but that didn't take away my sorrow for all she was missing. At the end of my father's life, he and my mother existed in their own private world, just the two of them. I don't remember her saying anything to me or to Ron. We were left to process our father's death on our own, certainly not as a family, and the only difference for me was that, instead of that sparking anger in me, I felt only grief for this family that had traveled through life in such separate orbits.

※

GENERALLY, IN THE support group, there were two approaches to the inevitable death of a loved one with dementia. People would either say something like, "They're so healthy physically, they'll probably outlive me. I think they'll live for another twenty years." Or they would react to how out of reach their loved one was and interpret that as death moving in fast. No one was ever right in their predictions. Death moves in according to its own timetable, and the one thing you can count on is that it will almost certainly surprise you. The other universal aspect of death is that when it does finally whisper that it's time now to say the last goodbyes, it's as if a giant mirror has been moved in front of you and almost every part of your life will be magnified. Death brings life into focus; it slips many things out of the shadows even as its shadow is descending.

I have heard people say that they didn't expect their loved one to die when they did, that they had just visited them and they seemed to have energy for more life. Often people wonder if they missed some sign, some behavioral clue that might have suggested the end was close. But that's trying to take ownership of something we can barely get our heads around. Death isn't ours to predict. That's not our job. Our job is to be fully open to the experience when it happens.

I have also heard people speak about warnings from doctors or caregivers at a facility, observations that their loved one is fading, and it might be time to make sure that plans are in place. They do exactly that, making all the appropriate arrangements. They find themselves jumping a bit each time the phone rings, thinking that this is when they'll get the news. But time rolls on.

That's what happened with my friends Cara and Thomas. The owner of the small nursing home where Michelle was living called them and said that he believed her time was short. She was declining physically, which Cara and Thomas had noticed the last time they visited, and all the signs were pointing to the end being near. Cara sprang into action, wanting everything to be set before her mother passed, so she could focus on her emotions without the pressure of making funeral arrangements.

She went to Pierce Brothers Westwood Village Cemetery, where many of entertainment's notable figures are buried, including Marilyn Monroe. Her mission there was to get a casket and arrange transportation of her mother's body to a cemetery up north where Michelle already had a plot next to Cara's father. Cara was about to get a crash course in the elaborate lengths some people go to after a life has ended. At the support group, after her visit, she reported how she had parked near Merv Griffin's burial site, where the inscription on the tomb reads, "I will not be right back after this message." She then described the unusual themes and coffins people can choose for their burials: a canoe-shaped coffin for avid canoers; a Western theme for a wanna-be cowboy or cowgirl (spurs on the coffin?). She had us all laughing, which is always welcome in a support group that gathers for a very somber and difficult purpose. I remember reflecting on how vital it is to make laughter a part of the dance between life and death. There is a line in an old Joni Mitchell song, "People's Parties": "Laughing and crying, you know it's the same release."

It took some time, but Cara and Thomas got all the arrangements made—a plain coffin, no theme, and a car to drive her mother's body north when the time came. Then they waited for the time to come. It seemed for a while as if waiting crowded out everything else. When they visited Michelle, the idea that time was growing short was always there, looming in the background. Then, something unexpected happened. Michelle rebounded, got stronger, and telegraphed that she probably wasn't going to be leaving them anytime soon.

More than two years later she passed away. Cara was greatly relieved that she had made all the arrangements beforehand because she was surprised at the depth of her grief, at the pain that swelled up in her even though she had prepared herself for the end for a very long time. But that's how it is with death—you don't know how you're going to feel.

❧

I WASN'T COMPLETELY PREPARED for how overwhelming my grief would be when my father died. After ten years of mourning as I watched him fade and move farther away into some misty realm that only he could inhabit, I thought I had gone through most of my grief. But the finality of someone no longer being here pulls the ground out from under you. You're in free fall, and though you will land, there are moments when it doesn't feel like you ever will.

A lot of things die with a person's passing. Like hopes that we still harbored: I have listened to other people talk about their secret wish that a parent would express pride in them or apologize for the wrongs and slights that had accumulated over a lifetime. That wish stayed lit, like a child's birthday candle, right up to the moment of death. Others have longed for a moment of recognition—the forming of their name, or a look in the eyes that said, I know who you are. We don't admit to ourselves how fervently we have been holding onto these hopes, because our rational minds have always suspected they would never materialize. But when death comes, we can't avoid seeing the wishes and longings that have dropped from our grasp. That becomes part of our grief, too—the empty space of our loved one's absence, and the weight of unrealized hopes.

Often, people in the support group would ask if they could still come once their loved one had died. I not only said they could, but encouraged them to keep coming because the grieving process was going to take them down unfamiliar paths. They would need the support that the group offered. I can say unequivocally that no one reacted in the way they once thought they would. People who believed they would not be overcome with pain were devastated. People who thought they would fall apart found a serenity they didn't know they possessed. Just as dementia is unpredictable, so is death and the reaction to it. Death, like dementia, will teach you valuable lessons if you get out of the way and let it.

As with everything in the world of dementia, there are differences when it's a spouse or a life partner, particularly with early-onset Alzheimer's, when someone way too young is facing death. The person who is losing their partner, their best friend, is haunted not only by life's unfairness, but also by the past—that bad argument years ago when things were said that shouldn't have been, the achingly tender things they never got around to saying, the plans they'd made for next year, but next year didn't look the way they had expected. Accepting death can be particularly wrenching in this situation. I've heard people say that you never get over it, but you get through it.

Losing someone close to us changes us forever. That's especially true if we are losing the one person with whom we expected to share much more of life. I think you have to hold on tightly to the richness of having known love that overwhelmed your heart, that defined your days and soothed your nights. Not everyone is that fortunate. With great love can come great sorrow. But that love is also what helps our hearts heal.

While I didn't have a support group to sustain me after my father died, I did end up finding comfort in an unanticipated way. The event of my father's passing and the services that followed were shared by the entire country. On the day of his death, the streets around my parents' house were almost impassable; people came and lingered. Days later, when we transported his coffin from the funeral home to the Reagan Library, which was the start of four days of services, people lined the streets and crowded onto freeway overpasses, waving at us as we passed. I felt, and still feel, that politics was left by the wayside for those few days, and that people showed up to mourn the passing of a good man, whether they agreed with him or not.

In an illogical way, I had resented America for its ownership of my father, even though it wasn't America's fault that he was elusive and hard to reach. But it was easier to blame the country than to accept that my father didn't want to be fully known by his children. So, it was ironic that, after his passing, America was functioning as my support system. The outpouring of sympathy and shared grief held me above the water line. I knew when it was over, I would have to sink down into the deep currents of my private grief, but for a while—for a few days—I could float above.

Years later, when I had the opportunity to help others in my support group, I could tell them from experience that, after the death of a loved one, being around others is vital. There will be time for solitude, there will be time to curl up alone with your emotions, your private thoughts. But right after a loved one dies, you need support. I'm not suggesting that you need the support of an entire country—that's a rather unusual circumstance. But find a few people to pull close, people who understand grief and loss, who are willing to be like arms beneath you, holding you up.

BY THE TIME the end comes, if you have surrendered to grief through the long passage of Alzheimer's, it might seem like there can't be much more of it left. After all, you've gone through the stages of grief many times over, you've lived with the unfolding of it in your life, you know its ebbs and flows. But when death comes, grief lets you know it isn't finished with you yet.

So much of how we grieve has to do with what our relationship was with the person who is gone. If the loved one you've lost is someone with whom you have had a difficult relationship, grief can feel like a strange dance. There might not be a lot you're going to miss if your history with that person was troubled and full of conflict. You feel the weight of loss, but it shifts, seems unbearably complicated at times. If that person is a parent who might not have been a very good parent, you've actually been grieving your whole life over what wasn't there. If instead you felt a bond with that loved one, then the emptiness that their passing will leave is something that opens up chasms inside you.

I've known both kinds of grief. Although my father was elusive and hard to know, he had a sweetness about him that made it impossible to resent him for his elusiveness. All his children longed to be closer to him, and missing him was woven through my life. As I got older, I realized how much being the child of an alcoholic affected him. He didn't have an available father, so how could he have learned to be one himself? I also realized that much of my rebelliousness and acting out when I was younger (and even into adulthood) was an attempt to get his attention. It usually worked, too. Getting in trouble, I learned early on, definitely got him to turn in my direction.

Many things passed between us in the Alzheimer's years; I felt, at the end, that forgiveness rested softly in the space between us. I had also finally come to know him a bit better. Stripped of memory and eventually cognition, his essence was left, and that essence was gentle and gracious. My grief throughout those years was infused with gratitude for having had the chance to see who he was at his core. It's the kind of grief that cradles you even when the tears won't stop, even when the heartache is relentless. The closest I ever came to bonding with my father happened in the years of his illness.

By contrast, as I have described, I had an extremely challenging relationship with my mother, and even when things were going well, I knew it was only a matter of time before they would splinter again.

I've spent decades unraveling the complexities of our relationship, and also grieving over the absence of a mother-daughter relationship in my life.

One evening in my support group, someone who had a tense and difficult relationship with a parent who had Alzheimer's confessed that they were afraid they wouldn't shed any tears when that parent died. It wasn't the way they wanted it to go down—they would prefer to experience the wash of grief that many in the support group expressed, but it didn't seem likely. I told this group member, rather than decide ahead of time what their reaction was going to be, to consider the possibility that they simply didn't know what feelings might arise. There might be deeper layers of grief there that they weren't yet aware of. Just be open to whatever comes up, I said, and whatever does come up will be the exact right thing.

That exchange resonated with me because it happened at the time when my mother was in the last months of her life. We knew how compromised her health was, and that it was basically a waiting game at that point. A part of me had similar thoughts to what this group member had expressed. How could there be any grief left in me? I knew I needed to listen to my own words and apply them to myself. When my mother died, it did feel different from my father's death—there wasn't the same sweetness or nostalgia. But then moments came when I would break down and sob. I was surprised that so much pain still came up from such a deep place in me, but I did what I'd asked other people to do. I surrendered to it.

The grief for a person you did not get along with can be far more difficult than mourning the loss of someone you were attached to. That's because the warmth, the softness, the fond memories that provide solace are missing. You are flung back into feelings of absence that are achingly familiar and have trailed you throughout your life. With my mother, I clung to the few memories I had of interactions that were loving and tender. I wasn't slipping into denial or trying to induce amnesia—we had the relationship we had, and it was not a nurturing one. But if I recalled those few times when something transported us past our differences, the moments when there was just love, my grief felt less punishing. I found myself feeling sympathy for my mother, for the fact that she never really experienced the joy of motherhood, that it always seemed like a burden to her. It gave me another dimension, softened some of the edges.

But there were still edges, feelings I didn't experience with my father's death. After he died, even though there were days that felt weighted, rife with sorrow, the overriding feeling was lightness, as if part of me had been pulled away from this world. I chose to think of it as a reminder that as human beings we don't ultimately belong here—we visit, for however long our life-span is, and then we go home. I imagined his soul tugging at me from the other side, just enough to remind me of that. There was a calmness to the time after his passing. The world around me seemed to be falling into step with my state of mind. I could have sworn that people were more polite in traffic, that no one was tailgating me or cutting in front of me. I know that probably was not the case, but it was my perception.

I vividly remember the day, about five or six weeks after his death, when I was driving and someone veered in front of me, causing me to slam on my brakes. I hit the horn, I yelled a few choice words, I probably flipped them off, and then I thought, "Damn, I'm back. I'm definitely not floating above the fray anymore."

In the weeks after my mother died, emotions blew in like storm winds through an open window. Emotions I thought I'd dealt with—had dealt with for so many years—in therapy, out of therapy, in prayer, in daily life—buffeted me. There was nothing gentle or tender about them. I'd been frightened of my mother all my life, and her death didn't magically remove that fear. And even though I searched my memory for times of tenderness, so many other memories intruded.

On the way to my parents' house, there is a curve on the road, about two minutes away, where my stomach would always clench. In the last years of her life, I visited my mother every week, sometimes more often, and every time at that same point in the road I'd feel my stomach grip with tension and dread. The morning I got the call that she had died during the night, I got in my car and drove over to her house. As soon as I came to that curve, my stomach clenched. I said aloud, "You don't need to be scared anymore. She isn't here." It didn't work, my stomach remained knotted up, and I realized that my mother had been such an all-consuming force in my life, I couldn't grasp that she was gone from this world. Even when I stood at her bedside looking down at her body, a part of me expected her to pop up at any moment and tell me to cut my hair.

It took almost two weeks, as we were going through the process of cleaning out the house, for me to pass that spot on the road and not have my stomach tie itself into knots.

Our personal history has deep, stubborn roots. The emotional underpinnings of our relationship with a parent don't dissolve with their death. Just as our physical muscles have a memory, there is a muscle memory to emotions also. Fighting against that won't help. The best we can do is be willing to crawl inside those feelings, take them apart, understand that they had a place in our lives at one time, but they don't need to be there now.

I've noticed that with any version of grief—sweet or challenging—impatience can intrude. Suddenly there is a sense of, "Let's get this over with." I think it's a symptom of our society right now, that everything has to be instantaneous. I read once that in a bygone time it was accepted that the grieving process took a full year. There is something lovely about that—taking four seasons to process a loss. Now we expect others, and ourselves, to bounce back and go shopping a few weeks after a loved one has died. It's as if we regard everything, even grief, as a potato we can put in the microwave.

With dementia, the stretched-out version of grief that begins as soon as the diagnosis is made is especially foreign to us. We're not used to slowing down; this disease asks us to. Fighting it, trying to make it move faster, is in the end not going to work. It might mean having to assert yourself with some people, because not everyone will understand.

Very soon after my father died, the day after I had returned from a week of public mourning, with services in Washington, D.C., and California, when I was finally able to take some private time for my own grief, a friend called and said something like, "I hope you're feeling better and are past everything." She then asked me if I could go to her house that week a couple of times a day to feed her cats, because she was taking her husband on a surprise trip for Father's Day. I was stunned. Not only had I just lost my father, but I had been in front of the world for five days. I'd had no time to sit quietly with my own feelings, and Father's Day was around the corner—a poignant occasion for someone whose father just died.

I said no and pointed out that there are pet sitters who do this kind of thing; I believe I added some words about the grieving process, which went right over her head. She is not in my life now; as I've mentioned before, people you know will reveal themselves in times of illness and death, and often what they reveal is that they shouldn't be in your life. While it feels like an added wound to have to separate yourself from someone you thought was a friend at a time when you needed support, the idea that nature abhors a vacuum is applicable to our personal lives too. Someone else, usually someone who you didn't expect, will step in to support you to fill the empty space. Tragedies, illnesses, death all change the landscape of our lives in many ways, including our relationships. It's difficult to see relationships change, to see people you thought were friends fall away, but ultimately those changes are going to be for the better. At some point, we look back and understand that the people who didn't belong in our lives had to leave so that new people, who do belong, could show up.

❧

As I write this, daylight is breaking on the anniversary of my father's death. On this day fifteen years ago, damp billows of fog filled the streets as I drove to my parents' house just after dawn. The day remained overcast, the sky telling no time of day until early afternoon, when my father took his last breath. I was glad, when I woke up this morning, that the day was soft and overcast, that it felt similar to the day he died.

A friend asked me yesterday if this would be a hard day for me. I said, "No, it never is—it's a reverential day, a day when I try to stay centered and close to God. That's how I felt sitting at my father's bedside. Like God was in the room." On this day, I remember my father's back as we rode horses along oak-leafed trails at the ranch my parents owned when I was growing up. He always rode ahead of me, and

I was constantly trying to think of something to talk to him about that would make him turn around and look at me. I remember him tan and strong at the beach where we vacationed in the summers. Even though the later memories of him, frail and confused, and in the end confined to bed, remain, they are not what my mind travels to. This is what time eventually does with grief—it peels back the sadness, the ache, and leaves us remembering moments of beauty. The sorrow remains, but it's one layer of a more complete experience. Avoiding grief, trying to outrun it, is by definition a rather frantic effort. People who are most at peace with themselves, I've noticed, are those who can stand quietly in the presence of sorrow—their own and other people's—and accept that it's part of life's dance of shadow and light.

A friend once told me that she had cried out to her therapist about a particularly painful time in her life, "Why is this happening to me?"

"Because you're alive," he replied.

❧

WE'VE ALL FELT THE effects of grief on a large scale, beyond the boundaries of our own lives. I was eleven when President John F. Kennedy was assassinated; my world was fairly small then. But I remember noticing how people behaved differently with each other—more familiar, more tender. Five years later, when both Martin Luther King Jr. and Robert Kennedy were killed, I felt it more acutely. The country seemed to slow down, people took longer breaths. When 9/11 shattered our lives, we looked at strangers as if they were friends, and no one bothered to hide their tears. When Kobe Bryant died and the pain of loss was everywhere, for a short while some of our differences and political rancor lessened.

When I looked at the hundreds of strangers who had gathered along streets after my father died, many of their faces were streaked with tears. Others were solemn and wistful. I wished I could have told all of them how much their presence meant. It was as if I suddenly had a huge family.

A couple of months later, a woman said to me, about the aftermath of my father's passing and the sadness that rested like a soft cloud over the country, "We needed that." I knew what she meant. People came together to mourn. They set aside their differences, the chasms that otherwise seem to separate them, and they just allowed themselves to be sad over the passing of a man who led America for eight years. A man who made a difference in the world, whether you agreed with him or not. It's not possible that all those people who stood for hours waiting to see the funeral procession pass were Republicans. The beauty was that it didn't matter.

Grief can be the most healing thing in the world. It opens us up, it makes us reach out to others, it inspires us to not take seriously the differences that divide us. It makes us look at life with wonder, at death with respect, and all of it as a fragile dance of time.

"Then for each one of us the moment comes when the great nurse Death takes man, the child, by the hand and quietly says, 'It's time to go home. Night is coming. It is your bedtime, child of earth.'" —JOSHUA LOTH LIEBMAN, *Peace of Mind*

CHAPTER 19

After the End

My father's scent lingered in his room for eleven days—I counted. It faded during that time but was still detectable whenever I passed by to go into my mother's room. Sometimes I allowed my thoughts to wander and consider that maybe he was lingering, just to see how my mother was doing. I wasn't sure I really believed that, since he spoke of going home to God with a certainty anchored in faith. So, he was probably safe in the world beyond. The scent was just molecules in the air, but the idea that his spirit might be drifting around made me smile.

My father used to tell a story about sitting at his father's funeral service and suddenly feeling Jack's hand on him, stroking his ear; it was something Jack used to do when my father was a child. I loved that story. I tucked it away in my imagination, wondering if I would experience something like that with my father. Maybe he would give me some sort of sign after he was gone. To this day, I can't say he has.

The closest I came to feeling that he visited me was a dream I had a few days after he died. In the dream, we were at the Malibu ranch that defined so much of my childhood. It was a thick foggy day and we were both on horseback. My father looked at me, shook his head sadly, and said, "There are so many things I got wrong. So much I need to be forgiven for." Then he turned and galloped away straight into a fog bank. I started galloping after him, trying to see him up ahead, but the fog was too thick. All I could see was white mist. I couldn't even hear the sound of his horse's hooves anymore. My father has appeared in other dreams of mine since he died, but that was the only one where I thought he might have been visiting me.

An actor friend of mine told me that after his mother died, he was sitting on the couch in his oceanside apartment with the sliding doors open to the sea. Suddenly a white dove flew in, perched on the couch next to him and stared at him with calm eyes. He was certain it was his mother. At that moment, his aunt called and told him that a rerun of his appearance on the Carol Burnett Show was on, so he turned on the television. As he described it, "My mother and I sat on the couch and watched me on Carol Burnett's show, and then when it was over, she flew away."

The point of these stories is that unpredictable things can happen after a loved one dies. So stay alert. And maybe set aside any preconceived ideas—just be open to whatever comes up. Death doesn't end a relationship, so whether you believe that departed souls can visit, or you just think that the imagination travels down strange roads in the midst of loss, it's a good idea to pay attention.

Not too long after my father died, my mother told me that she had several times woken up in the late hours of night and he was in her room, sitting on the edge of the bed. I was fascinated by this, and

I asked her how old he was, what he was wearing. My mother was not very detail-oriented, but she said that my father in these visits was not the age he was when he died. He was younger, and he was wearing, according to her, "regular clothes," which I assumed meant what he wore around the house or when he went to the ranch. The visits went on for a while. One evening, he was sitting in an armchair and she thought he looked cold, so she got out of bed and put a blanket around his shoulders.

I advised my mother to keep these experiences private. Many people don't believe in such things so, while I was very curious and interested in my father's visits, others might have a different reaction. She didn't take my advice, which is the only reason I'm writing about it. Had it stayed between the two of us, I would have kept it to myself even after her passing. But, for reasons I don't understand, she went public. One of the many people she told was Billy Graham. When she told me that she had spoken to Rev. Graham on the phone and had told him my father was visiting her at night, my first thought was that he was actually a good person to tell. But she looked quite crestfallen when I asked what his response was: she said that Rev. Graham had been dismissive, almost patronizing. According to her, he said, "Well, Nancy, I'm sure it makes you feel better to think that Ronnie is visiting you, but there is nothing in the Scripture to support something like that."

I was incredulous. "What?" I said. "I think there's a very famous story in the Scripture about exactly this. Jesus died on the Cross, and three days later, he was back on the road."

"Oh, that's right," she said, mulling it over. Unfortunately, I don't think my words carried the weight of Billy Graham's, and I wish I could say that her disappointment in his response made her more reticent with other people about these visits, but that wasn't the case.

I hope this will serve as a cautionary tale. Choose carefully whom you share information with. Whether you have a sense that your loved one is nearby after death, or is visiting you in dreams, or is even whispering to you sometimes, keep it to yourself or choose a confidant whom you trust completely, who will not discount or dismiss what you are telling them.

We are incredibly vulnerable after a loved one dies. What people say to us, or don't say, can cut deep. I will always remember the people who reached out to me after my father died, and I will also always remember those I considered friends who never reached out at all. I am aware that their silence was more wounding because I was so raw, but that's what death does—it peels away our protective layers.

One of the unique aspects of losing a loved one to dementia is that you think, during the years of their illness, that you are becoming accustomed to their absence. After all, they are not who they once were. They don't fill up the same space, they don't participate in life in the ways they once did. To some degree family and friends move on without them. Birthdays, holidays, graduations, marriages—these events all take place without them in attendance. But when they die, you suddenly realize that they were, in fact, taking up a lot of space. The emptiness of my father's room tugged at me whenever I passed it in the hallway. I understood then how much it had become the center of my parents' house. My father didn't take part in the life of the household anymore, but his presence was huge, even when he was confined to a hospital bed.

❧

OUR HISTORY WITH THOSE of us who are left to grieve doesn't die when the loved one does. All the feelings we ever had for them—good and bad—remain with us, taking up space for the rest of our time here. If we're lucky, we learned from them. Much of what I learned about my father came after Alzheimer's started stealing him away. I saw parts of him that he wouldn't have let me see on his own—the boy he once was, the lanky athletic teenager, the young man who looked beyond the flat landscape of the midwest to city lights and lofty goals, who decided he had a destiny to fulfill and it was on the world stage.

At a certain point, memories of your loved one before dementia take over and become most prominent. You may not believe that at first. The recent pictures are too vivid—a parent or spouse or sibling whittled away by dementia, looking out with distant, sometimes haunted eyes. How can those images ever fade? But there is a movement to grief. It shifts our memories, rearranges the images in our minds. In time, the most prominent will be of healthier times. These won't completely remove the memories of illness, but they can muscle them out of the way. I've heard it many times now—people confirming that, as months passed, the uncomfortable memories moved aside and older, better memories surfaced.

When my father comes into mind, I see him tall and strong, mounting his horse and taking off across wide fields to sail over jumps he and the ranch hand built from old phone poles. I see his eyes bright and blue as he talked to me—his young pudgy daughter—about leprechauns and enchanted forests, about heaven's sloping hills and clean waters. He stopped telling those stories when I got older and he, I suppose, deemed them too childish. What he never knew was, at an age when I shouldn't have wanted to hear about such things anymore, I still longed to. I see him counseling me on how to ignore bullies when a boy at school was frightening me and I was pretending to be sick so I could stay home. I see him glistening with sunlight and seawater, waiting for the wave that would give him the perfect ride to shore. I never see my father in his public roles, as governor and president, although that part of his life is inescapable. But those images don't rise to the surface when my thoughts turn to him. That was his public life, his other life. I have trouble finding my father when I look at him in those contexts. He returns to me as the man whose hands could fix anything and whose footsteps in the house made me feel that things would be okay.

I spent my life looking for a home, because ours didn't always feel like one. It was only after my father died, when I could reflect back on the ten years of Alzheimer's, the ten years of losing him in pieces, that I was able to say, this was always my home. Sometimes our homes are built with shadows and missing pieces. Sometimes there are rooms that are never unlocked. In the season of grief after he was gone, I realized that I needed to accept the imperfections and mysteries of the life I was born into. The reason I had learned so much from the years of his illness, from sitting beside him in both soft conversations and complete silence, was that I wasn't looking for anything beyond what the moment could show me.

Among all the lessons that Alzheimer's taught me, the lesson of acceptance towers above everything. The Serenity Prayer says, "God grant me the serenity to accept the things I cannot change." Alzheimer's taught me to stop fighting against what couldn't be changed and to ask instead, "What can I learn from this?" I didn't fully realize how profound the lessons were until after my father died, when I could look back and see that everything I had gone through was like a baptism. I would never be who I was before Alzheimer's came into my life.

I don't know why we are born to the people we're born to. I don't know why some people get a disease like Alzheimer's while others don't. I don't ask why anymore. I ask what I can learn. When I was small, my father told me I didn't have to stand on my tiptoes and reach up to the sky to find God—He is all around, He is always close, my father said. I wish that earlier in my life I had accepted that gift of wisdom.

A long time ago I followed my father out into the ocean, into deep water, to wait for waves that would carry us back to shore. Many years later, when we were both much older, I tried to follow him again as tides carried him out toward horizons that weren't mine to visit. I ended up floating in deep waters as he moved farther and farther away. Memories, regrets, hopes drifted around me, but it was the faith he had instilled in me that kept me from sinking. The people who live in our hearts never leave, even when they move on. Even when they die.

In 1994, a disease my family knew very little about descended on our lives and it seemed as if it would change everything. It was relentless and tyrannical—an unmatched pirate. But as years passed it became clear that Alzheimer's couldn't steal what the heart holds tightly. Sometimes sorrow and loss are our greatest teachers. We lose pieces of our loved ones when Alzheimer's claims them, but we also find them in unexpected and mysterious ways. Most importantly, we can find pieces of ourselves that were waiting for us.

Sometimes I walk along the beach in the early morning. I listen to the gulls, the crashing of the waves, and I imagine what it would be like to have my father walking beside me. I imagine his footsteps sinking into the sand and how he would probably be glancing out at the water, judging the waves to see if they were good for bodysurfing. I feel sorrow wind its way up inside me until I remember that he imprinted me in the deepest parts of my soul. It took years and a devastating illness for me to realize that, but once I did nothing was ever the same.

"All mankind is of one author and is one volume. When one man dies, one chapter is not torn out of the book but translated into a better language."   —JOHN DONNE

Afterword

One night in 2011 I woke up at three in the morning. A storm had blown in. Rain was raveling the tree branches outside my window and there was no other sound except the storm. I don't know if I dreamed it and then woke up with the idea, or if it came in with the rain, but I saw myself running a support group for people who were losing a loved one to Alzheimer's. I got up, went on the computer and looked for Alzheimer's support groups, just to see how crowded a field it was. Not very—I found only a few.

Before the month was out, I was sitting in Dr. David Feinberg's office at UCLA Medical Center, describing what I wanted to do. David Feinberg is one of those rare people who listens, and listens intently. Under his stewardship, UCLA Medical Center was devoted to making patient welfare the top priority. By the end of our meeting, I knew my support group had found its home.

For the five years that I ran the group at UCLA, I always knew he had my back. I was naïvely unaware that hospitals, like most establishments, can be brutally competitive and quite political in nature (not blue/red politics, but the workplace version of politics). When David left UCLA for Geisinger Medical Center in Pennsylvania, I found out quickly how valuable his protection had been. I have to admit I was blindsided by some of the betrayals that suddenly confronted me. But keeping Beyond Alzheimer's going was the most important thing. Since it was clear it no longer had a home at UCLA, I moved the group to Saint John's Hospital in Santa Monica. I will always be grateful to Dr. John Robertson for making that happen, and to Kate Johnson and the Deane F. Johnson Alzheimer's Research Foundation for helping me raise funds to keep it running.

In 2017 I had to make the difficult decision to end the support group. I had been running it twice a week for six years and was spending a lot of time researching facilities and day-care establishments, as well as looking into other things that came up in the group. My work as an author was piling up behind me. I had published one novel during the time I was running the group, but my next book was sitting woefully unfinished on my computer. I was also trying to put a documentary together, but not finding the time. Added to that was the reality that, once we moved to Saint John's, I had to run the group on donations. UCLA had funded the group when it was there, but that was not the case at Saint John's. No one is ever charged to come to Beyond Alzheimer's, but there are costs involved. I decided to work on licensing the program to hospitals.

On many occasions I have run into a sad realization that some hospitals don't see value in helping caregivers. Fortunately, Geisinger Medical Center in Pennsylvania and Cleveland Clinic in Las Vegas were exceptions, and Beyond Alzheimer's has been licensed by them.

I still hold out hope that more hospitals will see the importance of offering support for the caregivers of people with Alzheimer's and other types of dementia, so that they don't become patients themselves from the stress of their experience. Caregivers need someplace to go where they can talk, vent, cry, and even laugh sometimes. I have always felt strongly that Beyond Alzheimer's belongs in hospitals; that's typically where the frightening diagnosis of their loved ones is made, so it should also be a place where caregivers and family members can go to help heal themselves.

One of the hard realities of the coronavirus pandemic is that family members have not been able to visit their loved ones who have dementia and reside in facilities. They aren't able to be there as the disease steals more and more of the person they love. They aren't able to be there at the end. This has made an already painful situation even more excruciating. Which means even more people are in need of support and emotional sustenance.

I always emphasized confidentiality in the support group, and I have done my best to honor that in this book. In recounting certain stories, I have omitted male and female pronouns and used "they" instead, with the intention of blurring who I might be referring to. I have also blended some stories that were similar to make the points I was trying to make. In one specific story, as I made clear, I changed the names of friends who allowed me to use their story; their alter egos are now Cara and Thomas.

I will always respect and admire everyone who attended the support group during the years I was running it. They are some of the bravest people I've ever met. I learned valuable lessons from them, and I hope the group helped make their journeys smoother.

It's through challenging times that we grow and it's through times of grief that we learn to cherish joy—often the joy found in small moments and in events that might have seemed inconsequential at other times. My father's illness set me on a path to share those revelations with others who found themselves staring at the reality of dementia.

I've listened to enough stories now, counseled enough people, to know that dementia doesn't have to destroy the lives of caregivers. It's a difficult path, and at times it seems like there is no path, just darkness. That's when you need travel buddies. That's when you need other people who will hold out a hand and say, "Here—turn this way. You'll be okay."

Acknowledgments

I am grateful to Bob Weil and Gina Iaquinta for responding to this book in its infancy and for the wise and poignant editing (thank you for catching my occasional mixed metaphors!).

I will always be indebted to David Feinberg for his support for Beyond Alzheimer's. Thank you to my cofacilitators at UCLA—Linda Ercoli and Xavier Cagigas. To Hala Fam, thank you for your support and guidance. And at Saint John's I am grateful to Katie Mayo, Adam Darby, and Shereen Tabibian for cofacilitating and sharing their wisdom. Thank you to Carole Garcia for filling in sometimes. Thank you also to Kate Johnson and the Deane F. Johnson Alzheimer's Research Foundation for jumping in to help, and to Dr. John Robertson and Paul Mamulolous for giving Beyond Alzheimer's a place to meet.

Thank you to Dr. Bruce Miller for advising me on portions of this book and answering all my questions so promptly. And for their friendship, support, and love: David Rambo, Michael Reagan, Nikki Valko, Chip and Vicky Goodman, Donald and Andrea Goodman, Suzanne Simonetti, Lloyd Grove, Max Boot, Leo Mavrovitis, Paddy Calistro, Scott McCauley, Paul Sand, Reggie Sulley, and Michael Georgiades.

Notes

The World Just Changed

1. William Kreisl, Can a Smell Test Sniff Out Alzheimer's Disease?, www.cuimc
   .columbia.edu/news/can-smell-test-sniff-out-alzheimers-disease, March 28,
   2018.
2. Scott Gottlieb, Head Injury Doubles the Risk of Alzheimer's Disease, ncbi
   .nim.nih.gov, November 4, 2000.
3. Mayo Clinic, Anesthesia, surgery linked to decline in memory and thinking,
   sciencedaily.com, July 19, 2018.
4. Owen Gleiberman, "Robin's Wish" review, A Wrenching Look at Robin Williams' Last Days, variety.com, September 1, 2020.
5. Jennie Erin Smith, In a Colombian Family's Dementia, a Journey Through Race
   and History, undark.org, May 27, 2019.
6. The woman whose brain staved off her family's Alzheimer's, MIT Technology
   Review, technologyreview.com/2019/11/04/132061/the-woman-whose-brain
   -staved-off-her-familys-alzheimers/.
7. Bill Whitaker, Frontotemporal Dementia, Devastating, Prevalent and Little
   Understood, cbsnews.com, September 5, 2019.
8. Dr. Bruce L. Miller, *Frontotemporal Dementia* (Oxford University Press, 2013).

9. University of California, San Francisco, Nicholas Weiler, Lifestyle Choices Could Slow Familial Frontotemporal Dementia, eurekalert.org, January 7, 2020.

10. Cindy Chang, "Elderly Driver Who Killed 10 is Sentenced to Probation," nytimes.com, November 21, 2006.

11. Mayo Clinic Staff, Meditation, https://www.mayoclinic.org/tests-procedures/meditation/about/pac-20385120.

12. Elisabeth Kübler Ross, *On Death and Dying* (Scribner, 2014).

The Early Stages

1. Death with Dignity Acts, deathwithdignity.org.

2. Paula Span, "One Day Your Mind May Fade. At Least You'll Have a Plan," *New York Times*, nytimes.com, January 19, 2018.

3. JoNel Aleccia, "She Was Diagnosed with Dementia. She Documented Her Wishes for the End. Then Her Retirement Home Said No," *Washington Post*, washingtonpost.com, January 18, 2020.

4. Helen Schucman, Bill Thetford, Kenneth Wapnick, eds., *A Course in Miracles* (Foundation for Inner Peace, 1975).

5. Alzheimer's Association 24/7 helpline: (800) 272-3900.

Messy Emotions and Learning to Lie

1. Gavin de Becker, *The Gift of Fear* (Dell, 1998).

2. "The genetics of Huntington's Disease," Huntington's Disease Association, hda.org.uk.

3. Joe Dispenza, *You Are the Placebo* (Hay House, 2014).

4. Annette Kondo, "Blinding Horrors: Women's Vision Loss Linked to Sights of Slaughter," *Los Angeles Times,* latimes.com, June 4, 1989.

5. Alvin Powell, "When Science Meets Mindfulness," *Harvard Gazette*, news.harvard.edu, April 9, 2018.

6. Coleman Adult Day Services, What Is Sundowner's Syndrome?, colemanadultday.org, November 10, 2018.

7. Ken Keyes, *The Hundredth Monkey* (DeVorss and Company/Vision Books, 1982).

8. Norman Cousins, *Anatomy of an Illness* (W. W. Norton, Twentieth Anniversary ed., 2005).

9. Lavanya Ramanathan, "Lifestyle Guru B. Smith Has Alzheimer's. Her Husband

Has a Girlfriend. Her Fans Aren't Having It," *Washington Post*, washington post.com, January 28, 2019.

10. B. Smith and Dan Gasby, *Before I Forget* (Harmony, reprint ed., 2016).

When Things Get Out of Control

1. National Adult Protective Services Association, napsa-now.org.

2. Andrew Capehart, What to Expect When Working with Adult Protective Services, eldermistreatment.usc.edu, January 4, 2016.

3. Pamela D. Wilson, What Does Guardianship of an Elderly Parent Mean? pameladwilson.com.

4. Kamilia S. Funder, Jacob Steinmetz, Lars S. Rasmussen, Anesthesia for the patient with dementia undergoing outpatient surgery, 2009, ether.stanford.edu.

5. Tracey Tully, "After Anonymous Tip, 17 Bodies Found at Nursing Home Hit by Virus," *New York Times*, nytimes.com, April 15, 2020.

Rebuilding Your World

1. Joan Biskupic, "A New Page in O'Connors' Love Story," *USA Today*, abc news.go.com, February 18, 2009.

2. E. J. Mundell, "Love in the World of Alzheimer's," *HealthDay News*, abc news.go.com, March 23, 2008.

3. Jack E. Othon, *Carl Jung and the Shadow: The Ultimate Guide*, highexistence .com.

The End Stages

1. See getpalliativecare.org for an explanation of what palliative care is and more.

2. See Hospice Care, medicare.gov.

3. Caroline Richmond, "Dame Cicely Saunders," July 23, 2005, ncbi.nlm.nih.gov/ pmc/articles/PMC1179787.

4. Sogyal Rinpoche, *The Tibetan Book of Living and Dying* (HarperCollins, 1992).